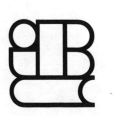

Creating
the New
American
Hospital

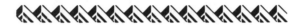

V. Clayton Sherman

Creating the New American Hospital

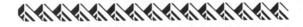

A TIME FOR GREATNESS

Jossey-Bass Publishers · San Francisco

Substantial discounts on bulk quantities of Jossey-Bass books are available to
corporations, professional associations, and other organizations. For details and
discount information, contact the special sales department at Jossey-Bass Inc.,
Publishers. (415) 433-1740; Fax (415) 433-0499.

For sales outside the United States, contact Maxwell Macmillan
International Publishing Group, 866 Third Avenue, New York,
New York 10022.

Manufactured in the United States of America

10% POST
CONSUMER
WASTE

The paper used in this book is acid-free and meets the
State of California requirements for recycled paper
(50 percent recycled waste, including 10 percent
postconsumer waste), which are the strictest guidelines
for recycled paper currently in use in the United States.

The ink in this book is either soy- or vegetable-based and during the
printing process emits fewer than half the volatile organic compounds
(VOCs) emitted by petroleum-based ink.

Library of Congress Cataloging-in-Publication Data

Sherman, V. Clayton.
   Creating the new American hospital : a time for greatness /
V. Clayton Sherman.
     p. cm.—(The Jossey-Bass health series)
   Includes bibliographical references and index.
   ISBN 1-55542-514-3 (alk. paper)
   1. Hospitals—United States—Administration. 2. Organizational
change. I. Title. II. Series.
   [DNLM: 1. Hospital Administration—organization & administration—
United States. 2. Hospital Planning—United States. WX 150
S553c]
   RA971.S485 1993
   362.1'1'068—dc20
   DNLM/DLC   92-48943
   for Library of Congress   CIP

Credits are on p. 311.

FIRST EDITION
HB Printing   10 9 8 7 6 5 4 3 2   *Code 9312*

THE JOSSEY-BASS
HEALTH SERIES

Contents

Preface

In each age men of genius undertake the ascent. From below, the world follows them with their eyes. These men go up the mountain, enter the clouds, disappear, reappear. People watch them, mark them. They walk by the side of precipices. They daringly pursue their road. See them aloft, see them in the distance; they are but black specks. On they go. The road is uneven, its difficulties constant. At each step a wall, at each step a trap. As they rise the cold increases. They must make their ladder, cut the ice and walk on it, hewing the steps in haste. A storm is raging. Nevertheless they go forward in their madness. The air becomes difficult to breathe. The abyss yawns below them. Some fall. Others stop and retrace their steps; there is a sad weariness. The bold ones continue. They are eyed by the eagles; the lightning plays about them; the hurricane is furious. No matter, they persevere. They stand on top of the world.

—Victor Hugo, *Les Misérables*

It is the best of times in health care. We have reached levels of supersophistication in medical practice, pharmacology, and technology. We are rapidly achieving better distribution of health care in terms of outpatient, home care, and preventive services. The promise of genetic engineering is on the immediate horizon. Medical knowledge is doubling every five years. We are literally on the verge of being able to deal successfully with hundreds of problems we were powerless to deal with before. It is a time of miracles.

It is the worst of times in health care. Costs are wildly out of control, quality of care is often horrific, and ethical problems abound. Health care has priced itself out of the market for increasing millions, and the quality is less than that available in other nations. Regulations are chaotic, anachronistic, even stupid. Health care workers are deserting the field in droves. Customers are mad. Hospital presidencies turn over at alarming rates. It is the worst mess the industry has ever suffered — a time of disaster.

The hospital industry is undergoing revolutionary and needed change. The old cost reimbursement model has been replaced with the oncoming shock waves of a much more wrenching and uncertain future for the industry. The hospital is an increasingly difficult organization to manage. There are incredible forces to be dealt with, and they are not being managed well.

Why This Book?

The *bad news* is that time for managing change is running out. Hundreds of hospitals have already closed their doors, yet too many hospital leaders have hunkered down, hoping these changes will blow over. They won't. Organizations that do not adapt quickly may find that their window of opportunity has completely closed.

The *good news* is that a crisis period is the best time for a book such as *Creating the New American Hospital*. As recently as 1985, very few hospitals understood the problem as one requiring complete organizational renewal. Today, nearly all of them understand the need for change. That understanding is a key ingredient for energizing each hospital and mobilizing its key players.

The purpose of this book is to give to all those who can be leaders for fundamental change in the American hospital an outline of how to achieve such a transformation. The challenge is to convert their organizations from their present maladapted state to the future organizational archetype that I have called the New American Hospital. This book is designed to provide answers to two major needs that executives must deal with in creating the New American Hospital: first, a clear picture of what the New American Hospital is and how it should be managed, and second, a plan for managing the change process. This is a road with many turns and oncoming hazards that are hard to discern. The journey is arduous, and the labor and effort to make the trip will take the best we can give.

The book details what the New American Hospital should be like in its management approach, use of people, response to the Customer, organizational structure, and creation of market-valued innovation. I have chosen to capitalize the words *Customer* and *Associate* (employee) wherever they appear in the book. This is to acknowledge their central importance to the organization's functioning and to symbolize my profound respect for them. Words denoting members of management are left lower-case to indicate their servant role to both Associate and Customer and to lessen internal status differences of an organization. These concepts are more fully developed in later chapters. The capitalization style I have chosen serves to illustrate in a small way the radical break the New American Hospital makes with the old.

The book spells out in considerable detail the how-to's that must be incorporated into the way things work in hospitals. We know enough now about what an excellent organization is and how it works to apply these principles to the specifics of the hospital industry. An old argument held that the principles of organizational management did not hold for the "special case" of the hospital industry. That argument, specious at best, no longer is true in today's increasingly difficult and competitive world; it is a false view that will crumble as past ideologies are bulldozed by economic reality and market requirements.

Hospitals have much to learn from the best of American organizations and from successful corporations around the world. It is time to understand that past governmental financial support arrested organization development and prevented management excellence. The dole of government intervention held up the development of quality, service, and innovation. The industry needs fewer handouts. It needs greater understanding of how to create a high-performance hospital.

None of these statements is a criticism of past leadership in the industry. From the 1930s through the 1980s, hospital leaders built an industry that provided America with a tremendous standard of health care. The history of these executives' careers is one of great contributions. Under the rules of the game that applied in those decades, hospital leaders played the game well and achieved considerable success. But the rules have changed, and winning now requires that the approach to the game also be changed.

Can executives who are successful in a noncompetitive environment learn new competitive management approaches? Can organizational leaders who learned management in a noncompetitive world successfully master the entrepreneurial realities of a free market? These questions remain to be answered in organization after struggling organization. One certainty is that leaders who adapt themselves to the new management approaches outlined in this book will stand the best chance of successfully harnessing the forces at work in their organizations.

Will the model work? Emphatically yes! The major portion of what is written here has been implemented in nearly one hundred hospitals that are doing well. Indeed, it is their story that I recount, their successes and failures and the lessons learned along the way. These New American Hospitals are not perfect in their performance, but they have fostered stronger cultures, have much-improved business results, and enjoy happier Customers and more motivated workers. They represent examples of success, and where they compete head-on with an old hospital, they prevail. Their quality is better, their speed is faster, they function more smoothly, and they gain the market share that such performance deserves. Other hospital organizations can learn much from them. Answers are at hand — answers that have been tested in hospital environments and found to work.

Who Should Read This Book?

This book is for today's health care leaders at all levels — hospital presidents and other members of top management, department managers and supervisors, boards of directors, medical staff, health planners, and others responsible for the redirection of the industry. On their capable shoulders falls the challenging, wonderful opportunity to create renewed organizations and a better health care future. It has been my great privilege to work with leaders who reflect the passion and willingness to give themselves in a worthy cause, to pay the price excellence requires. To those who are willing to lead, this book gives not only the strategic direction that wide-scale change needs but a whole host of specifics to make it possible.

Those who read this book will adopt some pieces, adapt others, and from their own creativity extend and expand upon these ideas. The reality of any management situation calls for wisdom and tailoring, not the simpleminded following of a rule book. It would please me as an author to have readers of this work tear it apart, debate it, and sift through it for ideas they deem useful. The book is a departure point, a frame of reference. But it is also a comprehensive picture of a problem arena that has too often been subject to cosmetic and piecemeal approaches. It is my desire that all who are interested will borrow liberally from it. The job that needs to be done is great, and there is little time.

While problems abound, there are even more solutions. In every case of my work with hospitals, I have found that the managers, and the dedicated people who work with them, have always known what needs to be done and have always shown their willingness to roll up their sleeves to do the work.

This book is also for employers, insurance companies, government agencies, and private citizens, all of whom are tired of paying the bill for management inefficiency and uncertain quality. This book is also for students and faculty of health care administration, who are responsible for reconceptualization and expansion of knowledge in this critical field—they will be an important bridge to the future. Finally, and most importantly, this book is for patients, families, and physicians—all the Customers of the hospital. One overrriding consideration that has guided me in writing *Creating the New American Hospital* has been my concern that we create an organization that is worthy of these folks. We *can* do a better job for them all. We must.

How the Book Is Organized

The book is divided into three parts. The first, "Building a Brighter Future for American Health Care," argues that both the cause and the cure of hospitals' failure lie with the leaders of America's health care organizations. Rather than continuing to endure the endless list of troubles that America's hospitals suffer, it's time to build the kind of future that is needed. To accomplish that, management must first change how they run the organization.

Chapter One, "Why Hospitals Fail," details the argument that most of the cost, quality, patient dissatisfaction, and morale problems with which hospitals are besieged are caused by mismanagement— not primarily because of bad managers, but because of discredited practices that have ruined other industries as well as our own. This management philosophy is bankrupt, and so too are the organizations that follow it.

"Reinventing the American Hospital," Chapter Two, puts forward the notion that hospital executives and managers can cure many organizational ills by changing their approach to management, Customers, and Associates. To accomplish this, both a personal management renewal and an organizational revitalization must be achieved. The task is arduous, but it has been implemented in a number of hospitals that are now reaping substantially better managerial and organizational performance.

Part Two, "How the New American Hospital Functions," describes the differences between old and new approaches to Associates and Customers as well as to the work, management, and organizational structure. The new model parallels the best practices found in America's foremost companies and shows how they can be applied in a hospital setting.

Chapter Three, "Unleashing People for Contribution," describes how the New American Hospital reverses the ways people are thought of at work. This chapter identifies a number of tragically inept uses of people that must be eradicated and then lists prescriptions for dealing with people in a positive way. Outmoded personnel practices that suppress talent must be cleared away, but ridding the organization of these practices will not be enough. There must be a whole new approach that utilizes the amazing strengths that people have. With no increase in salary costs, it is possible to make tremendous gains in worker ideation, motivation, productivity, and quality.

"Delivering the Service Strategy," Chapter Four, shows that attacking Customers' problems requires far more than training in guest relations or responding to complaints in a reactive fashion. The New American Hospital approaches Customers' needs strategically, putting together all the needed elements, rather than just following a fragmentary approach. The value of this chapter is that it gives a picture of a more comprehensive and coherent solution than the single programs hospitals have implemented, and it shows how the New American Hospital pursues its Customer service strategy in the broader context of managing the rest of the organization's needs.

"The Quality-Productivity-Innovation Equation," Chapter Five, examines how the new hospital gets work done. Rather than focusing on only a Total Quality Management program, New American Hospitals know they need to look at a wider range of interlocked objectives to become more efficient. Fortunately, many solutions and many answers can achieve these ends. Quality-productivity-innovation enhancement cannot be achieved in the old hospital. Organizational renewal is the only certain way to achieve it.

Chapter Six, "A Streamlined Management System," details how managers need to follow the effective approaches to management that have been profiled among the best men and women in the profession. This involves establishing a system of management that can significantly change organizational results by revving up problem-solving quality and speed, streamlining operations, and creating a healthy climate that fosters risk taking and innovation. Until managers perform differently, the organization will not perform differently.

Chapter Seven, "Optimizing Organizational Structure," shows a number of ways to rethink the deployment of people at work. There is no ideal organizational structure, but by changing the design of the organization, people often get a lot more done—or feel as if they want to. This chapter focuses on how changing the organizational chart and formalizing relationships can act as a support mechanism for the more important changes occurring in the New American Hospital.

While the previous part describes how the New American Hospital functions, making the transition from old to new becomes the real trick. In the final part, "Succeeding in Organizational Renewal," I share the change management approaches developed in many brave hospitals over the last decade. I try not only to present the principles that must be followed in leading wide-scale change, but to give a number of specific applications that spell out the various pieces and phases of this process. The model is one of rapid renewal.

"Leading the Transition," Chapter Eight, shows that to create a New American Hospital there must first be a new approach to hospital leadership. This requires changing how executives and managers do their job, and how they then lead the transformation effort. Only then can Associates change the way work systems affect Customers. This chapter details a radically different approach to managing the enterprise, describing what leaders have to do to manage organizational change successfully and to lead people through the change process. It is a profile of winning managerial behavior.

"Managing Wide-Scale Change and Reconstruction," Chapter Nine, is outside the experience of most hospital executives. Neither they nor department managers have ever dealt with managing an organizational transformation. This chapter presents the elements that must be managed successfully to control rapid and major change. Renewal managing is a big jigsaw puzzle that can be successfully put together, but all the pieces, and how to put them together, have to be understood, planned for, and executed with precision. The chapter concludes with an overview of how the organization development process is structured. Look here to get a quick snapshot of how the changeover is accomplished.

Chapter Ten, "Preparing for Transformation," shows that organizational change follows a sequence and requires a rigorous battle plan. This chapter focuses on the first wave of the change process. During the *preparation wave*, the necessary work of conducting organizational assessment, achieving executive "buy-in" and support, and arranging coordination to launch the effort is accomplished.

Chapter Eleven, "Implementing the Renewal Strategy," is an outline of how to undertake the major work of transformation that occurs in the first year during the *implementation wave*. This model should be considered a general outline, a working approach to changing the hospital from the old to the new form. This is the most complex and difficult phase of the renewal campaign.

"Accelerating the Change Process," Chapter Twelve, is essential to maintaining the changes that were accomplished during the implementation wave. To some degree the *acceleration wave* evaluates, consolidates, and refines the gains made thus far. But this is also a time to institutionalize changes so that the organization doesn't slip back, a common problem that undermines much organization development work. Accelerating and refining the change process challenges people all over again and completes the transformation.

"Driving Change with Rewards," Chapter Thirteen, is an approach that keeps change on track, makes it fun, and keeps the organization driving forward. The New American Hospital plays into human greatness by setting up the system so that doing the right things pays off, for both the Associate and the organization. It brings a host of new recognitions, reinforcements, and rewards into being to help sustain the change effort, and it removes old hospital paradigms that reinforced wrong behaviors and supported the status quo.

Can our hospitals be transformed into organizations of excellence? Each who would lead must look in the mirror and answer that question. It is a time for greatness. For our children, and for our place in history, it is time to build the New American Hospital. It is time to attempt the climb up to the mountaintop.

Style of Writing

As a professional communicator, I know how difficult the writing process is, and how easy it is for the audience to be turned off, especially when the message is as challenging and difficult as the one in this book. I apologize to any who might be offended by messages that are confrontational concerning the way things are managed in the industry now. I do not want to lose a single reader. Instead, I invite you to be open to this challenge. I believe deeply in today's health care leaders, but I do not believe that success will come from some of the obsolete ideas that were passed along to them. My criticisms aren't personal; they are conceptual and practical. Use the ideas in this book to win — don't fight them and lose.

Gender usage in this book alternates between male and female pronouns to indicate that the examples and situations described are nonsexist. It is a fact that there are still too few female and minority executives and managers. Nothing in this book is meant to perpetuate an image of leadership as being a limited domain.

Finally, my writing voice reflects the frankness of my personality. I tend to say things directly, and I am guilty of using analogies to sports teams or the military that not everyone cares for. Because I am writing as a consultant practitioner, my voice is sometimes first-person — this doesn't mean that my experience is the source of all wisdom, just that I am reporting my experience. I do not apologize for any of this; I simply beg for the reader's understanding of my limitations.

Acknowledgments

Where does one begin to express appreciation for all who helped? Sir Isaac Newton once said, "If I have seen further it is by standing upon the shoulders of giants." Certainly this is how I feel. I am most indebted for the ideas and many stories in this book to my clients. It has been a privilege to serve them and an education to learn from those who carry the heavy burdens of running America's hospitals. What crazy and grand people they are! When I first asked whether they thought it would be worth the risk to try to implement the management ideas found to work in other industries, they laid their careers on the line and risked their very organizations. What vision that took, what courage! Each succeeding organizational changeover resulted in dozens of alterations in the working model that is presented here. My clients' experience in the field wrote this book.

I am indebted to many beloved professors and to the work of countless researchers and academics. My struggle has been to implement their ideas and, to my delight, find that they work. I will never forget reading *In Search of Excellence* — it gave me the "Eureka!" experience, for it articulated my own observations and provided a beginning point for the model that is now set before you.[1] My limited contribution has been to translate ideas and to blend different perspectives. Many others have invented the ideas that are the ingredients I have attempted to assemble into a hearty recipe for hospitals. Where I have been able to give attribution I have done so, and a lengthy list of suggested readings is appended at the end of the book.

I wish to thank my wife, Stephanie, for her willingness to give up weekends and nights. Her ideas as colleague, helpmate, and loving supporter are all in this book. My special thanks to my other Management House colleagues — John Hilliard, Judy Kopp, Debbie Paddock, Jan Salerno, Amanda Soukup, and Ken Weidner. These special people contributed and challenged, have been my friends, and did my work while I wrote this book!

A special professional thanks to Rebecca McGovern, my editor at Jossey-Bass. Her ability to balance criticism and at the same time give encouragement kept me writing and made this work possible. At times it has been a labor of love; at other times, far less than that. At about the seventh revision, Alis Valencia, editor of *At Work: Stories of Tomorrow's Workplace*, got involved as a reviewer and suggested many organizational changes.[2] Her fresh outlook added much to streamline the flow.

Inverness, Illinois V. Clayton Sherman
January 1993

Notes

1. T. J. Peters and R. H. Waterman, *In Search of Excellence* (New York: HarperCollins, 1983).
2. A. Valencia, *At Work: Stories of Tomorrow's Workplace*, Newsletter published by Berrett-Koehler and Designed Learning, Cazadero, Calif.

This book is dedicated to my mother and the memory of my father.
Their example of achievement, vision, and perseverance
taught me that we must choose and create the future we want.

June M. Sherman

Commended by the president of the United States
for pioneering efforts with the mentally ill. Her favorite saying:

I think I can, I think I can, I think I can.
— Watty Piper

Vernon W. Sherman

Commended by the Department of Defense for contributions to the
war effort and the building of the atomic bomb during World War II.
His favorite saying:

Nothing will ever be attempted
if all possible objections
must first be overcome.
— Samuel Johnson

The Author

V. Clayton Sherman is founder and president of Management House, Inc., Inverness, Illinois. Management House provides management development, organization development, and human resource services to a wide range of Fortune 500 companies, hospitals, associations, and emerging growth organizations. He received his B.S. degree (1966) in psychology from Brigham Young University and his M.B.A. degree (1968) in management and Ed. D. degree (1975) in management development from Western Michigan University. He has also done post-doctoral study in managing organizational effectiveness at Harvard University's Graduate School of Business and studied with W. Edwards Deming in the area of quality improvement.

Sherman's primary consulting experience concerns itself with wide-scale change processes and organization renewal. He specializes in hospital revitalization and high performance management. His work has won the Best Video Conference award sponsored by the National Association of Video & Satellite Networks. One of Sherman's clients received the 3M Innovations in Health Care Award for the organization's transformation using the New American Hospital model. He serves as a keynote speaker for major conferences in the health industry including the MacEachern Lecture at the Congress of the American College of Healthcare Executives.

Sherman's audiocassette programs, "The Uncommon Leader" and "Strategies for Stress Free Living," have been among the best-selling management programs of all time. He is also author of several books, including *From Losers to Winners* (1987) and *Managerial Performance and Promotability* (1984). Prior to his entry into consulting in 1978, Sherman was corporate director of human resources for Upjohn Healthcare Services, Inc., where he was responsible for a personnel complement of 70,000 and winner of Upjohn's Award of Excellence.

Part One

BUILDING A BRIGHTER FUTURE
FOR
AMERICAN HEALTH CARE

1

Why Hospitals Fail

I dare you. I double dare you. I triple dare you.
— America's playgrounds

This chapter explores how the management assumptions, systems, and approaches used today have led to an industry in crisis. It is now becoming clear why hospitals fail and why they will have to be radically changed in order to succeed. Indeed, what is needed now is the birth of the New American Hospital, a revolutionary new form of hospital organization that can both improve quality and control costs, even in the current unworkable operating environment. What's needed is a new American revolution to transform hospitals into what they need to be for the twenty-first century. This book is designed to help leaders make that transformation.

The story of the New American Hospital is a success story. It is neither fantasy nor fairy tale, but an account of a daring journey taken by a growing band of courageous hospitals. It is a story of battle, of warfare over ideas, and of a fight to win the hearts and minds of Customers and staff. It is a story of difficulties and some defeats. And it is a love story, a story of dedication, risk, and the achievement of a promised land. The legend is a blend of *Rocky, Atlas Shrugged*, and the *Odyssey*. Here, now, is the story of how to win in running America's hospitals.

The story begins, as good stories must, with trouble in the kingdom.

An Industry in Crisis

An endless litany drones on in the nation's press about the troubles of the hospital-centered health care industry. A brief

3

synopsis of its symptoms shows why a new hospital form is needed:

- Mired in a system in economic crisis, afflicted with market myopia, and regulated beyond sense, American hospitals are either closing their doors or cutting services.
- Lawyers circle in an ever-greater feeding frenzy over the issues of medical malpractice and quality.
- Key professions such as nursing can't find students to fill their classrooms, and turnover levels surpass those of most other industries — painful testimony to mounting disaffection.
- The economic impact of health care costs has become devastating to the national economy, with a financial meltdown predicted. Calls for national health insurance only raise the question, "Why fund a failing system?"
- American business is having to cut benefits to workers, deny coverage to the retired, and cancel retirement benefits to cover health costs. Executive choices are not pretty. What's the alternative? Bankrupt American business to feed a failing health care industry?
- Individual pain leads to emotional stories of people caught in the maelstrom of canceled coverage and personal bankruptcy caused by health care costs.
- Even at a premium price, the quality of patient care can be well below acceptable levels. Sometimes care is world-class, sometimes far less.

Clearly, something isn't working.

Why Hospitals Fail

Organizations fail because of poor management. Studies show that in other industries, executives often blame all sorts of external factors — labor attitudes, costs, or governmental regulation — for their inability to compete, in much the same way that too many hospital executives believe that the magic answer will be found from some outside source such as national health insurance. But while external problems in these industries don't make it easy to do business, they have not been found to be the cause of decline. Robert Hayes's blockbuster analysis of American industries showed that an organization's failure to compete has little to do with economic, governmental, cultural, or labor issues. *It is primarily a failure of management.* He said, "The conclusion is painful but must be faced. Responsibility for this competitive listlessness belongs not just to a set of external conditions but also to the attitudes, preoccupations, and practices of American managers. By their preferences for serving existing markets rather than creating new ones and by their devotion to short-term returns and 'management by the numbers,' many of them have effectively forsworn long-term technological superiority as a competitive weapon. In consequence, they have abdicated their strategic responsibilities."[1]

Management's failure to do all that it can internally to offset external problems is usually found to be the primary causative factor leading to defeat. This is a continuing problem, a failure that persists for lack of recognition. More than a decade after Hayes's findings, W. Edwards Deming said, "The kind of management being practiced in American corporations now and being taught at American business schools is the biggest producer of waste, causing huge losses whose magnitude cannot be evaluated or measured. Most people in management are not aware that they are imprisoned by current practices of management. . . . that these management practices are the cause of American corporate decline. [These practices] prevent companies from functioning efficiently as a system."[2]

Is it possible that hospitals are failing now because of improper management? Regina Herzlinger's analysis was stinging in "The Failed Revolution in Health Care—The Role of Management":

> The American health care industry is sick. . . .
> Americans find services to be fragmented, impersonal, inconveniently located, and offered at unsuitable times. Then there is the quality of the care itself, which is notoriously erratic. . . . In response

to demand and to the perceived inadequacies of
the system . . . a revolution [occurred] in the 1980s
that was supposed to transform the health care
picture.

But the revolution failed. . . . What went
wrong? I claim that the failure was almost entirely
that of management, not of strategy, that the
creators . . . were so blinded by the vision of the
dazzling new world they hoped to forge that they
neglected the details of management that would
breathe life into their vision.[3]

This analysis sees a failing system, a needed revolution, and a
management that is not attending to its task. Specifically,
Herzlinger accuses executives of pursuing marketing and financial strategies, but showing *managerial neglect*.

But is it really fair to blame management for the ills the
hospital industry is suffering? Wouldn't these problems have
been cured by more money from a rich Washington Uncle? An
article in *Modern Healthcare* maintains that this is not true: "Low
Medicare and Medicaid payments didn't close 81 hospitals last
year, a link espoused by hospital industry executives and swal-
lowed whole by the media. . . . The blame in many cases should
be placed on hospital executives who waited too long to respond
to changes in their market. . . . *Poor management likely was responsible for at least half of the hospital closings last year* [emphasis
added]. . . . Despite changes in their markets, many troubled
hospitals wait too long to adapt to those changes. . . . The
hospitals hesitate to make operational changes, such as cutting
costs, or strategic changes, such as altering services."[4] The
accountability, and possibility, lies with management, not in
hoping for a more ideal operating environment.

The natural inclination in a crisis is to find somebody to
blame. Yet there isn't a better-motivated or harder-working
group than those who run America's hospitals. We're not going
to get very far in the reforms that need to be made if all we do is
point fingers. The magnificent women and men who struggle
each day to provide the nation's health care aren't to be

blamed — they've done a wonderful job, healed a lot of people, and saved many lives, all within a climate where mere survival as an organization is a miracle. No, it isn't the people who are to be blamed, but the system of management that is producing poor and insufficient results. The challenge now is to find those who will accept accountability to improve the system.

The buck stops on the executive desk and with each member of the management team, no matter how much some would like it to be otherwise. And while it may not at first be apparent or believable, the hospital industry's problems are less a matter of fixing external factors than of doing what's needed internally. This book profiles case after case of hospitals that have changed how they manage and are thriving in the present hostile climate. These hospitals provide the hard evidence of the power of this thesis, their voices the chorus of the industry's future.

Hospitals everywhere are being buffeted by the need to adapt to market requirements and are besieged by economic starvation. It is "do or die" time, and the continued failure of health care organizations suggests that more dying than doing is going on. Why don't they change?

Hospitals do not meet new demands because they have not improved their basic capability to process change, structure new work relationships, and develop a coherent organization. They fail to show the adaptive capacity needed in turbulent times, and what results is a disjointed effort to meet this need. At its very root, the American hospital industry suffers from mismanagement and insufficient leadership at all levels. Hospitals fail because of an obsolete approach to management, not because of financial problems or competition. A new approach to management is needed, not new managers — if they will accept the accountability to find that new way.

The solution doesn't lie in national health insurance or in passing along increasingly higher costs. Today the challenge isn't to fix what's wrong with the hospital, but to create a new kind of hospital. This New American Hospital, like everything else America has created, isn't going to be a slight revision of somebody else's ideas. It will be cut from new cloth and will break the mold.

JCAHO Is Not the Answer

The Joint Commission for the Accreditation of Healthcare Organizations (JCAHO) has reaped a whirlwind of criticism for ignoring the fact that accreditation is not an effective approach to quality control. Indeed, the whole question of why an anachronism like the JCAHO even exists needs to be dealt with by the industry as it turns to higher standards for the future. Pulitzer Prize–winner Walter Bogdanich, widely known in the business community for his understanding of quality control issues, exposed this issue and fanned the controversy by writing *The Great White Lie: How America's Hospitals Betray Our Trust and Endanger Our Lives.*[5] As *USA Today* wrote: "Walt Bogdanich . . . lays bare the hospital industry's dirty little secrets: waste, greed, incompetence — plus enough bureaucratic arrogance to rival the Kremlin in its salad days. 'It is a system built upon . . . a myth holding that hospitals and doctors are equally good and deserving of our complete, unquestioning trust,' he writes. 'That such a belief should still prevail in our country is as disgraceful as it is dangerous.'"[6]

It's important to see in all of this two essential arguments: first, that quality cannot be controlled by outside regulators and only competent internal management can get at the source of quality problems and second, that the denial of management problems by some in the health care industry will no longer stand. We are now at a point where the criticisms are so severe that there is nothing to hide behind. It's time to change.

The accountability, and possibility, lies with management, not some external group. This was vividly expressed by John White, then president of Floyd Memorial Hospital in New Albany, Indiana, as he took over a dying organization in 1985. In a speech to his management team, he challenged them with these words:

> What's all this nonsense of being in fear of the JCAHO visit? Do you mean that you're going to run

around like chickens with your heads cut off to clean everything up just to pass what JCAHO itself refers to as "minimum standards"? Then that means that we have been providing service at less than minimal levels. That's just not good enough.

We're not here to follow standards. We're here to set standards. The last thing we should be worried about is whether we can meet standards set by a bunch of outsiders who don't know what you do, and who don't have any responsibility for your patients. Let's be very clear about this. We have one standard and it applies to every department, every person, and every piece of work that we do. That standard is excellence. And anything that is less than that standard is to change, starting now.

By 1987, two years later, his hospital was rated best in Customer-satisfaction surveys, showed a rapidly growing market share, and was outpacing its competitors. Success clearly lies in a land far beyond that envisioned by outside regulators.

The Birth of the New American Hospital

The old hospital is so causative of its own problems, its management approaches so discredited, that nothing less than its death and complete replacement will produce the changes the market requires. Twenty-first-century health care will not be delivered by a management system borrowed in the 1930s from American industries that have long since been destroyed by others using smarter approaches to managing work, serving Customers, and releasing the power of their workers. The old management approach of the American hospital doesn't work, and it's not worth saving. Let's state it strongly so the point is clear: *a totally new direction for management is now required.*

What is needed is a New American Hospital. The New American Hospital is so unlike the old hospital that it would be almost unimaginable by executives of an earlier era. Its birth is being led by a new breed of executive whose primary contributions are an innovative set of assumptions and the committed energy to carry them out. These assumptions are that the Customer is king, that empowered Associates ("employees" in old hospital terminology) have the brains and will to deliver what the Customer requires, and that the first piece of business is to completely destroy the old "nonsystem" in favor of a new management machine.

Understanding the Ways of Change

The exciting news is that the management model described in this book has been tested and is now working in numerous American hospitals, and that a way out of the crisis is at hand. The book is about the experience of hospitals who are succeeding by having done all that I will write about. It tells in great detail their stories of how they made high-performance organizations out of struggling hospitals.

As hospitals try to improve, they need to focus primarily on creating a new kind of management system and organizational model that will serve as the foundation for all other improvement efforts. To accomplish this, managers must first master their craft and learn how to play like a team. They then must go to work to clear away the underbrush of old policies and systems in preparation for the work of building organizational excellence. Associates can then take over to accomplish the thousands of changes required in every aspect of the organization's performance.

The New American Hospital is not a panacea. It, too, has to deal with all the problems that exist in the industry. *But the first and most central issue on the hospital change agenda has to be a restructuring of its management approach.* Even when this managerial factor can't offset the damage done by other forces, it still creates an organization that is faster at responding, better at serving, more beneficial in motivating, and more protective of quality than any other type. What the New American Hospital management approach does is create an organization that thrives.

Periods of great change favor organizations that are quick

on their feet. In sports, the team with greater morale, training, and coaching talent tends to win. In battle, the army with the better strategy, newest technology, and more adaptive organization has better survival potential. The hospital that has these things often survives by picking up where the competing hospital suffers from maladaptation—not so much beating the competitor as being there when it fails to survive the assailing forces.

Stopping the Creation of Fear

Unfortunately, our hospitals are filled with fear and anxiety that occasionally approaches paranoia. People are intimidated, sometimes by autocratic and demeaning supervision, but more often by a system that seems out of control. Whatever the cause, it's certain that people will not embrace change, which is always fearful, unless the atmosphere in the organization is supportive and encouraging.

I don't think we have to drive out fear as much as we need to stop creating it. For too long, failing hospital executives have been sending messages of fear. Cost containment may be a legitimate issue, but the drumbeat of cut, slash, and pare are debilitating to morale. The threat of layoffs or liability lawsuits and the message that competitors are winning are not going to bring hallelujah shouts from the frightened. What lousy leadership this is.

Compare these leaders to Bill Gonzalez, who announced to his management team when he took over as president of Butterworth Hospital in Grand Rapids, Michigan, "We're not here to play defense, or to be ordinary, we're here to play offense, and to be extraordinary. We're going to be the best. We're going to do our best thinking and develop this organization—not for today but for the long term. We're going to be the premiere hospital in West Michigan. Let others worry about *surviving*. We're going to worry about *thriving*." Gonzalez understands the simple truth, that cost and competitive worries belong only to routine, mediocre organizations. You don't have to worry about secondary problems if you go on the excellence offensive. When you're excellent, there are no competitors. When you're excellent you've got volume and cash flow is not a problem. There is no guarantee that a good offense is the best defense, but that's the way to bet the business.

For some, the idea of going on the offense, of besting competitors and playing to win, is repugnant. Their sensibilities are offended; the idea that the achievement of excellence is a battle is distasteful to them. Everyone is entitled to an opinion, even when it's wrong. Perhaps it would help those who feel queasy if they realized that the New American Hospital intends to be the best, and *when it is the best, it will also be first*. Let those who don't wish to play to win explain that to their Customers. To do well in a competitive world is not to wish the competitor a bad day or organizational death. Excellence is a state of mind and attitude before it is a state of hospital performance. We simply intend to do our best, and we invite all others to join us, to run with us. Doing well in a competitive world doesn't mean that we can't work cooperatively. But we won't settle for the status quo or hold back the energies of our people.

As an industry, hospitals have often focused on the wrong questions. It was never cost containment that was needed, but productivity. It was never nurse recruitment, but nurse retention. It was never guest relations, but Customer service and system improvement. Similarly, the question now is not whether hospitals will survive, but whether they will choose to be excellent. When the culture is led by executives who proclaim that the organization is going on the offense, that it will attack across the entire excellence front, the organization receives a powerful, positive uplift, a total reconceptualization of the challenges that lie ahead. On the other hand, when old-time administrators frame the debate as one of survival, it creates unhealthy paranoia and the spirit of fear that is associated with losing.

New American Hospital executives are leading the charge, espousing this positive philosophy and putting forward the idea that doing our best *will* be good enough. This is leadership. Passing the test of that leadership means staying focused on the destination, not the difficulties and impossibilities of getting there or the voices saying we shouldn't take the trip.

A New American revolution is under way. It is a true

revolution in that it breaks the old paradigm. It requires a whole new conceptual base as well as new approaches to the messy work that revolutionaries perform. The reader will be jolted by what follows, for it challenges all the old assumptions and old ways of thinking. Yet this is not a theoretical treatise, as when Thomas Paine wrote of a revolution he hoped would come. The ideas and applications in this book work. Do these things, if you dare, and share in the success. You can bet your career on it.

Notes

1. Robert N. Hayes, "Managing Our Way to Economic Decline," *Harvard Business Review* (July–August 1980), pp. 67–77.
2. "Deming Still Produces the Quality of Belief," *Chicago Tribune* (December 29, 1991).
3. Regina Herzlinger, "The Failed Revolution in Health Care — The Role of Management," *Harvard Business Review* (March–April 1989), pp. 95–103.
4. "Why Hospitals Close," *Modern Healthcare* (March 24, 1989).
5. Walt Bogdanich, *The Great White Lie: How America's Hospitals Betray Our Trust and Endanger Our Lives* (New York: Simon & Schuster, 1991).
6. "Tale of Health Care Could Induce Nausea," *USA Today* (December 15, 1991).

2

Reinventing the
American Hospital

The cowards never started,
The weak died on the way.
Only the strong survived.
—Pioneer saying

It is hard to recognize when the past ends and the future begins, but we are living on such a hinge of history. It is difficult to admit that a former way of management in which we are proficient is failing now, but that is what brings us to this moment in time in which the American hospital must be reinvented, rethought, and rebuilt. This chapter will define the New American Hospital in terms of its deep service approach to Customers, its radical utilization of its people, and the efficient and machinelike way in which it gets work done. The chapter will discuss redirecting management operations and will show that there is an essential need to rethink the work objectives the hospital is to achieve and gain a firm grip on them to avoid the work drift that represents managerial malpractice in the old hospital. Perhaps the most difficult part of the reinvention is devising a change strategy and then figuring out how to carry it out. Fully half of this book is devoted to that problem. Finally, the chapter looks at sample results and benefits to be derived from building such an organization.

What Is the New American Hospital?

The future never just happens; it is created. Even though change and information are exploding, they aren't going to explode in

14

your organization unless you have an effervescent culture, and managers driving it who are skilled at assimilating and mastering change. There will be no twenty-first-century health care in our hospitals unless we learn how to birth it.

People will still get sick and need services, and so the American hospital will survive. But it will be transformed and will not be a hospital at all as we know it; what passes as acceptable quality today will be radically eclipsed by higher standards. It is not a question of whether there will be market demand, but for what, and when, and where, and at what level of cost. Today's generation of health managers is crucial, because epochs of change are epochs of greatness. These leaders will have to stop practices we're proud to have achieved in order to find something better.

Whether the hospital will even be called that in the future is anybody's guess. Already the greatest volume of service is done in outpatient areas and emergency rooms. The concept of the hospital as a central location where people check in for intensive care is already past, altered by new technologies, patient education, and distribution points of care.

As a collective term, the New American Hospital is not a location or a physical place, but rather a set of beliefs and practices about how Customers should be served, how Associates are utilized and motivated, and how the hospital should be managed. The prescriptions of the New American Hospital apply to extended care facilities, treatment centers, home health, and all organizational forms of delivering care.

The Associate

The organization is its people. But while the stated values of respect for life and the importance of people are given lip service in the old hospital, its practices toward its staff are not always consistent with that view. Job security has not been provided, abuse of staff is tacitly allowed, dissatisfaction and turnover are high, and employees are undertrained and underutilized, illustrating a belief that people can't do more or better than they do now. The old hospital believes that its biggest problems are financial and Customer service, and that is where program emphasis has been placed. The New American Hospital knows that the first priority is its people and the creation of a great place to work. Take care of your people and they'll take care of the Customers and the work. The comparisons that follow show how widely divergent are the views held about people at work.

Old Hospital	*New American Hospital*
Human beings referred to as:	*Human beings referred to as:*
Employees, personnel, full-time equivalents	Associates, Partners, Teammates
Subordinates, lower-level employees, hourlies	Prime competitive advantage
Disposable units of cost who can be laid off	Human resources whose jobs are inviolate
Job design and voice:	*Job design and voice:*
Paid to perform tasks	Paid to improve system
Time clocks and supervisory rating used	Time trust and self-governance followed
Individual accountability	Team accountability
Fixed jobs, step raises, and salary grades	Flexible hours and jobs, merit and incentives
People fit to jobs and organization	Jobs and organization fit to best people
Work role and voice:	*Work role and voice:*
Managers decide, workers implement	Semiautonomous work teams
Work piles up, continual stream of orders	Quarterly work planning
Information only on need-to-know basis	Information widely shared and available
Limited voice, paid listener-consultants	Wide participation and direct feed-in

Chapter Three provides a more complete view of the major shift in emphasis toward America's hospital staffs. They, and only they, have the talent, the will, and the answers to today's urgent need to change.

The Customer

The discredited control model of the old hospital has failed to satisfy Customer wants and needs. Customers are complaining loudly and litigiously about problems of quality, availability, and cost. But what can be done? As responsive executives and managers wrestle to find the answer, a whole range of new approaches are being tried. These are laudable as a first approximation to a solution, but as a complete answer, they are insufficient. The New American Hospital realizes that a successful reinvention of Customer-centeredness requires a radical philosophical and cultural shift, a major overhaul or replacement of existing work systems, and a comprehensive strategy that covers all of the needs of the hospital's customer constituencies. The following comparisons may serve to highlight the differences and distance between the old and new approaches.

Old Hospital	New American Hospital
Customer viewed as:	*Customer viewed as:*
Patients *or* doctors	All who benefit from what is done
Procedure name: gall bladder	Customer is king
Ignorant, "Who's the doctor here?"	Customer is always right
Intrusion, annoyance	Let Customer teach you your business
Quality and services approach:	*Quality and services approach:*
Defined by provider	Defined by Customer
Technology-driven	Market-driven and value-added
High-tech	High-tech, high-touch
Piecemeal programs	Comprehensive, from soup to nuts

Organizational orientation is:	*Organizational orientation is:*
Our policy requires . . .	What does the Customer require?
Turfs and departmental handoffs	Team, seamless performance
Conflict, find reasons to say no	Consultative, find solutions
Crisis-reactive, apologize for problems	Proactive, zero Customer defections

While the desire to serve the Customer is found in the old hospital, the absence of strategy, systems, and supportive culture makes it impossible to deliver service, at least at the level that the Customer now expects. Chapter Four outlines a detailed approach to altering these components.

How the Organization Is Managed

The crux of the problem lies in how the organization is missioned and managed. The old hospital has often lost sight of its values. Even though it holds endless conferences to rewrite its mission statement, it fails to implement the approaches that would achieve it. Its problem is not conceptualization of the goal, but poor execution of a work plan to reach it. The new hospital often has the same stated values as the old; the difference is that it lives them, carrying them out in every expression of its work life.

Old Hospital	*New American Hospital*
Mission strategy and emphasis:	*Mission strategy and emphasis:*
Make a profit, or slash costs by layoffs	Serve market, add staff for expansion
Make and sell	Competitively market position

Manage finances, cut deals	Manage "Wow" service, build great staff
Rely too heavily on financial measures	Measure all seven key result areas
Structure and control:	*Structure and control:*
Hierarchical, bureaucratic, top-down	Flat structure, teams, mutual influencing
Control through policy, rules, procedures	Value-centered management
High consultant usage	Associate and Customer input shapes business
Leadership style:	*Leadership style:*
Emphasis on authority, title, degree	Emphasis on results, promotion from within
Class prerogatives, status	Minimal status, first-name basis
Closed meetings, remote management	Hands-on supervision, managing by wandering about (MBWA), open meetings

Managing the quality-productivity-innovation equation (Chapter Five), creating a streamlined management system (Chapter Six), and optimizing the organizational structure (Chapter Seven) are elements that need to be dealt with in order to improve management of the New American Hospital. And there is a final factor. As leaders approach the task of reinventing the hospital (Chapter Eight), they realize that they cannot successfully change the hospital until they are willing to change what they do. A radical shift in managerial behavior is called for.

Changing Who Does What

To accomplish the changes that are envisioned, it will be necessary to change what people do, not just the situation around them. What does this mean for each of the following groups, and how will their roles be affected?

1. *Executives* move to the sidelines and focus on strategic and resource issues.
    *   Forced download delegation, fewer levels
    *   Increased executive control and managerial freedom via management by objectives (MBO)
    *   Executive approval times shortened to one to four weeks
    *   Collapse and consolidation of the organizational structure
2. *Managers* take over operations, executives do not make in-house decisions.
    *   Greater budgetary authority, fewer signatures, direct information sharing
    *   Intensive management development, socialization, and team bonding
    *   Reduced policy controls on managers
3. *Associates* are powered up.
    *   Semiautonomous work teams and wide participation in groups
    *   Skill and cross-training, collapse of job descriptions, people empowered to act
    *   Intensive upgrading of human resource approaches
4. *Customers* become kings.
    *   Customer councils, strategic Customer response, prime ideation source
    *   Customers rate quality, managers, and departments and partially determine rewards

By reducing the amount of vertical interaction required for communication and decision making, energy is redirected into the horizontal work flow of the organization. By deemphasizing vertical authority and emphasizing horizontal throughput, the organization operates with greater speed, gusto, and common sense.

Redirecting Management Operations

No one in American management has as tough a job as those who lead our hospitals. The complexity and importance of the job, the pressure and sheer volume of the work, and the challenges of running an applied science organization in a scary economic and political climate make this the toughest kind of organization to manage. How easy it is to lose sight of our objectives, to get distracted as we move from one crisis to another. To reinvent the hospital successfully, we must approach this problem by understanding how to monitor all necessary management tasks so that needed elements do not fall between the cracks.

Managerial KRA Deficiencies Equal Malpractice

Every manager in every organization has to achieve in seven key result areas (KRAs):

1. Customer satisfaction
2. Quality
3. People growth
4. Organizational climate
5. Innovation
6. Productivity
7. Economics

For a management team to be considered truly effective, all seven KRAs must be satisfied. To fail to produce results in any of these areas, whether as an individual manager or a management team, is to participate in *managerial malpractice*. This malpractice may be the fault of individual managers, lack of training, poor executive direction, or lack of system support. The old hospital fails to achieve many of its needed outcomes. Organizational malfunction is caused by managerial malpractice. Changing to a total KRA approach allows the organization to function correctly. But how can a management be sure it's doing the right things?

Keeping Your Eye on the Ball

Measure the right things to get the right results (Exhibit 2.1). When management measures the wrong things, or fails to mea-

Exhibit 2.1. KRA Goals and Measures.

Goals	Measures Type	Measures Indicator
Customer Satisfaction		
"Wow" service	O	Overall customer survey rating*
	O	# compliment letters/calls*
	O	Interdepartmental customer rating*
	O	Physician satisfaction rating
Response timeliness	O	On-time delivery (customer defined)
Zero defections	O	% of repeat customers
New services	O	% sales from new services
Preferred supplier	O	Share of key accounts' purchases
	O	Ranking by key accounts
Customer partnership	O	$ value of patient-submitted ideas*
	O	$ value of physician-submitted ideas*
	P	# patient-submitted ideas*
	P	# physician-submitted ideas*
	P	# cooperative efforts
Quality		
Zero defects	O	# standards violations/incidence reports*
	O	# complaint letters/calls*
	O	# of service "corrective actions" taken*
	O	# of lawsuits*
	O	Size of average claim*
	O	Clinical quality indicators best in market*
	O	Rework cases as % of patient activity
Best in class	O	Market survey ranking*
	O	Room and food service level (AAA, Mobil)
JCAHO standards	O	Pass JCAHO review*
People Growth		
Attract best people	O	% of positions vacant*
	O	Employer of choice ranking
		Candidates' ranking of employers
		General survey
Optimize use of people	P	# hours training/associate*
	P	Training as expense budget %*
	P	Promotions within/outside
	P	Total $/days of consultant usage
New learning	P	# inservice topics offered*
	P	% associates inserviced*
Keep best people	O	Turnover rate*
	O	# of disciplinary actions*
	O	Length of employment at turnover
	O	Position vacancy-related overtime
No subperformance	P	% of associates subperformance
	P	Individuals with action plans underway
Culture and Climate		
"Best place to work"	O	Attitude opinion survey*
	P	% new hires referred by staff
Living our values	O	Associate rating managers as excellent
	O/P	# policy/procedure improvements
	P	# culture hero awards

A fun place	O	% associates receiving performance awards
	O	% associates receiving attendance awards
	P	# department social events*
	P	# organizationwide social events*
	P	% departments with social events

Innovation

Wide participation	P	# of Do It Groups (DIGs)
	P	% associates making suggestions
	P	% associates involved in DIGs
High ideation rate	O	$ value of associate (non-DIG) ideas
	O/P	% intangible DIG improvements rated substantial
	P	# suggestions made*
	P	# suggestions/associate*
High implementation rate	P	% suggestions implemented*
	P	% DIGs implemented*
New service introduction	O/P	Introduction schedule vs. plan
	O/P	New service introduction vs. competition

Productivity

High output/input ratios	O	Full-Time equivalents (FTEs)/# adjusted occupied beds*
	O	Net revenue/FTE*
	O	Net revenue/associate payroll
	O	Net revenue/manager payroll
Resource efficiency	O	ROI$/DIG
	P	Average meeting rating
	O	% meetings rated lower than eight
	O	Rework estimate
	O	Revenue/$ of consumable supplies
Productivity technology	P	PCs/FTE
	P	$ for work tools (fax, photocopy)
Service excellence	O	Cycle/wait time/customer type*
	O	Unit cost/customer

Economic Benefits

Survive	O	Cash flow
	O	Expense control within budget
	O	Reduction in operating costs
	O	Return on assets
Succeed	O	Sales growth
	O	Net income
Prosper	O	Increased market share*

Type of Measures:
  O = Outcome measures. Measures that indicate whether you have reached the goal.
  P = Process measures. Measures that indicate progress on actions that contribute to outcomes.
* Indicates measures to be initiated during Implementation Wave.

Source: Management House. ©1992. Reprinted with permission.

sure the right things, it can never correctly control or direct the business. Most hospitals fail to measure managerial outcomes. New American Hospitals obtain good results because they work hard to control all of the essential areas of the business. While the organization doesn't fall into the trap of thinking that measures are results, it works hard to reinvent its measurement systems to parallel real program changes occurring within the organization as it undergoes renewal.

Identifying broad goals for each KRA, then establishing measures for each goal, are the first steps to gaining greater control over all of the hospital's desired outcomes. Measures of both process and outcome are needed, along with quarterly and year-to-date performance numbers. With these data in hand, it becomes possible to give directionality to the organization by setting targets for each goal. Finally, work initiatives that will help achieve KRA targets can be identified and worked into quarterly performance plans (see Chapter Five for a discussion of performance planning, a simple MBO system). Shown in Exhibit 2.1 are organization-wide measures, some of which could be applied to all departments. Usually, departmental KRA measures are more specific and represent a shorter list. The key is to provide the feedback to allow each leader to change whichever KRA isn't performing correctly.

This is the hard work of managing, the nitty-gritty of identifying goals, targets, and the work to be done, and then measuring to make sure it's been achieved. Yet it is this kind of tough-minded managing that is so notably missing in the old hospital. It is accurate to say that no hospital of the old type measures half of these items. Old hospital measures are often strongest in the economic area, for the financial people have usually done their job well. But the New American Hospital measures and then acts in all areas of needed performance, understanding the synergy and balance that must be achieved between the KRAs.

Creating a Change Strategy

Reinventing the hospital is a massive undertaking, a change management problem of such magnitude that few people have led such an effort. The implementation of wide-scale change in a complex organization can only be achieved by meeting three requirements for achieving excellence:

1. A sweeping overhaul in corporate culture
2. A radical shift in management philosophy
3. A permanent commitment at all levels to seek continuous improvements

Consider those words carefully: "sweeping, radical, permanent commitment." A little bit of change in the culture won't do it; this is a complete overhaul. Management assumptions and practices aren't going to change slightly; they will change totally. And finally, this won't be a temporary emphasis. It's designed for the long haul, involves everybody, and means challenging everything in the status quo. This is not a project for the fainthearted.

It's essential for members of the management team to think through the sequence and timing of the changes they want to make and the impact on people those changes will have. Part Three of the book represents one fully developed approach to doing that. Describing the changes that need to be made is easy; developing a change plan to pull it off is a bigger challenge. By way of briefest overview, elements of an effective change plan might include the following headlines.

1. Assess the corporate culture and history.
   - Does this model fit what your people believe and what your market wants?
   - Does the CEO have the desire, passion, and vision to lead major change?
   - Would executives be supportive and open to criticism and participation?
2. Create a battle plan for change. How will the strategy of change be implemented?
   - Think through the sequence, content, calendar, and sociology.
   - Set up coordination groups and processes to steer the change effort.

- What tactics will be pursued? What problem priorities will be established?
- Move early to minimize restrictions on policy, procedures, and authority.

3. Commit the generals, train the officers, and enlist the army.
   - Initiate major management development and redefine managerial roles.
   - Push forward against the status quo and problems.
   - Organize everybody in groups; involve a high percentage of people in the first year.
   - Zero in on team-building needs, socialization; add friendliness to the group.

4. Focus on the important issues.
   - Build the management machine; do away with the old system.
   - Remove Associate irritations early, stabilize job security, and rein in restrictive personnel practices. Begin longer-term development processes and job expansion.
   - Remove Customer irritations and begin moving toward zero defections. Make the Customer king.
   - Begin smoothing operations by attacking systems, quality, and productivity problems.

5. Deal with change elements and problems.
   - Kill off old hospital restrictions; demonstrate the new culture.
   - Drive with values, measurements, and rewards.
   - Blur the chain of command, set up new structures, and control the clan agendas.
   - Pursue symbolic wins and quick fixes to set the tone; publicize victories.
   - Heavily market internally, use intensive communication to reduce confusion.

6. Initiate new measurement systems to monitor changeover and establish reward systems to drive it.
   - Run periodic audits and attitude-opinion surveys. Ask, "How we doin'?"
   - Install a KRA measuring system and tie it to managerial rewards.

- Restructure the compensation package and reward schemes to drive change.

But what happens if all of this change work is done and nothing happens? Suppose that an organization takes the risk to make this changeover only to come up short in results?

Results in the New American Hospital

Effective leaders are not wedded to any philosophy, management concept, or change program unless it produces results. Effective leaders think in terms of what is practically attainable, not of an ideal that is impossible to achieve. The model of the New American Hospital described in this book isn't smoke and mirrors — it exists now. And it can be replicated elsewhere when leadership and the power of will are present. This new hospital form works and produces predictable and substantial benefits. Hospitals that have reinvented themselves typically achieve KRA outcomes like the following ones, which are drawn from many hospitals:

1. *Customer satisfaction*
   - Customer satisfaction ratings ("Service received was above average or excellent") increased from 78 percent to 92 percent in one year.
   - Market share increased against competitors by 19 percent in three years.
   - The ratio of customer complaints to compliments dropped 76 percent within twelve months after the onset of renewal.
2. *Quality*
   - Lawsuits and threatened legal actions dropped 50 percent in the first year.
   - Quality standards violations dropped from sixty-five per month to fifteen per month after one year of change effort.
   - A problem-solving team changed the radiographer notification procedure using flowcharts to optimize re-

sponse time and decrease operating room staff waiting
by 75 percent. Similar reductions in wait time were
achieved throughout the hospital.

3. *People growth*
   - The turnover rate dropped from 21 percent to 4 percent
     in two years, a pattern not common to the surrounding
     labor market.
   - Nurse vacancies dropped from fifty to none in a tight
     labor market. An improved general reputation in the
     market as the employer of choice resulted in zero expen-
     ditures for recruitment advertising.
   - Hours of training doubled, and expenditures for train-
     ing increased 50 percent at no new cost, financed by
     demonstrated gains in error reductions.

4. *Organizational climate*
   - Employee opinion survey scores jumped in eighteen
     months from an average category score of 71 percent to
     87 percent.
   - Physician animosity was reduced drastically in the first
     year following the change effort. The president now
     spends zero time handling the few physician com-
     plaints remaining with managers who are now em-
     powered to handle them.
   - Hospital experience has been universal that managerial
     passive-dependent behavior ceases, replaced by a can-
     do attitude that keeps challenging the system.

5. *Innovation*
   - Employee suggestions jumped from 28 to 1,836 change
     recommendations per year in the first twelve months
     following New American Hospital conversion.
   - The suggestion implementation rate went from 10 per-
     cent to 65 percent in the first year, and to 82 percent in
     the second year.
   - A hospital met its goal to implement 1,000 small-group
     change recommendations in twelve months.

6. *Productivity*
   - Net revenue per salary dollar increased from $2.10 to
     $2.40 in two years, a 14 percent increase.

- Net revenue per full-time equivalent (FTE) went from
  $50,450 to $57,664 (an increase of 14 percent in one
  year) in one case; in another setting, it went from
  $51,082 to $63,533 (an increase of 24 percent over four
  years).
- A hospital opened a large building addition with forty-
  three additional FTEs but no increase in overall costs
  due to productivity improvements.

7. *Economics*
- Revenue went from $51.1 million to $80 million, up 56
  percent, with expenses increasing from $30.4 million to
  $44.6 million, up 46 percent, and net income up $3.2
  million over a period of three years. In a tougher second
  case, revenue increased $17.3 million, while expenses
  increased $16.2 million, with net income up $1.1 million over a two-year period.
- A hospital went from a $5 million annual operating loss
  to $650,000 profit in twelve months due to worker par-
  ticipation efforts, with no loss in jobs.
- A hospital had a sustained record of increased sales and
  profits for each year since organizational revitalization
  seven years before.

Can We Get Similar Results?

*Caveat: The New American Hospital model will not work everywhere or
under all conditions.* While committed organizations have been
able to achieve tremendous results, their output was possible
only because of the change effort they put into it. Not every
organization has the leadership, talent, or will to work for
these gains.

As you consider the chapters in Part Two, you will see in
greater detail how such an organization must be managed. This
picture may be so foreign to your own institution that you will
think it impossible to achieve. In Part Three, you will see how the
reinvention change process is engineered. Again, this may be
frightening or impossible to achieve in your organization. *Because of the difficulty of the task of reinvention, some hospitals should be*

discouraged from even attempting it. It has been our experience that even where there is buy-in to the philosophy and practices of the New American Hospital, some organizations simply are not able to handle the implementation. In such cases, the hospital should postpone change until needed elements can be put in place. Ask yourself: Could our team do this? Are we enough of a team? Do we have the will, the time, the energy?

Some organizations will never start this journey. For them, the destination seems foolish or impossible to reach. Others will fail in the effort, unable to put together the many elements required or lacking the skill to manage powerful resistance to change. Only the strongly courageous, hardworking, and envisioned dreamers will succeed.

Part Two

HOW THE
NEW AMERICAN HOSPITAL
FUNCTIONS

3

Unleashing People for Contribution

It becomes perfectly true to anyone who will think this thing
through that there is no such thing in a [work setting] as
Management and Men having different functions or being
two different kinds of people. Why can't we think and why
don't we think that all people are Management? Can you
imagine any president of any factory or machine shop who
can go down and manage a turret lathe as well as the machin-
ist can? Can you imagine any manager of any organization
who can go down and manage a broom—let us get down to
that—who can manage a broom as well as a sweeper can?...
Obviously, all are Management.
                                    —James Lincoln
                    Founder of Lincoln Electric Company[1]

People are the most important change element in organizational revitalization. But to enlist their willing support and
creative energy, the dead weight of old personnel practices must
be removed, and there must be an end to demeaning employeeism that resides in the old hospital. It is important to go back
to the basics of good selection and training, along with a new
approach to structuring jobs and defining what people are
allowed to do. Finally, in an industry beset with layoffs, we need
to rethink how the problem employee population can be reduced and provide job security to those who perform.

The Primacy of People

The phrase "Power to the People" is redundant. That's where the
power always lies. Today we hear a lot about "empowerment," a
concept where management gives power to Associates. What
managerial conceit! What really happens is that management
finally gets out of the way of the people, and lets them do their

work the way they want to do it. Empowerment is a decision by management to stop *depowering* people. The old hospital is run by a management that thinks of power as a zero-sum game — there's only so much of it, and it has to be concentrated at the top by denying "permission" to others and requiring endless authorizations and committee reviews. How tiresome, and how out of touch.

"Knowledge is power" is irrevocably true today. Today's hospital management often supervises technical people with a knowledge base that top management can only dimly comprehend. The Declaration of Independence says, "That to secure these rights [life, liberty, and the pursuit of happiness], Governments [managements] are instituted among Men deriving their just powers from the consent of the governed."

True leadership derives its power from the willing delegation of power *to* the leaders by those who are managed. Only when they exercise "just powers" does the group dynamic really operate. What we see in the old hospital is a George III management, a legitimized coercion, that stops the flow of true power. It's time for a revolution!

The test question for any organization serious about achieving excellence is: *Does the organization fit what our best Associates need?* If not, change it! The first and best rule of thumb to follow in making changes designed to optimize human performance is to get rid of things that don't fit or feel good to the best workers in the organization. If your hospital is losing its best nurses, ask them why they're leaving. Believe what they tell you, and make changes to prevent such loss in the future. If people say they need more training, or day care for their children, or better equipment to do their jobs, do it.

A hospital is only a pile of bricks until people walk in in the morning. Yet it is amazing how this prime reality is forgotten, and how secondarily people are treated. The general prescription of fitting the organization to the people, instead of the other way around, pays off for the New American Hospital.

Reining in Restrictive Personnel Practices

Our experience with organizational transformation has shown that personnel policy and practice often acts as a major block to renewal and change. Stop this negative influence early in the game; it is a poor use of people that will also hamstring other changes that need to be made.

Removing Associates' Irritations and Grievances

As early as possible do an opinion survey among Associates. This invariably lifts the lid on all the unpleasantness that management pretends doesn't exist. For executives wanting to make a change it provides powerful and accurate information on exactly what's wrong, and it encourages managers to work out solutions that will be visible to their boss. Take away people's head-in-the-sand defenses, make Associates' needs a battle cry, and see the positive effects this has for the change effort. If you want the army with you, speak up for them!

Growing People, Not Administering Personnel

Management of people is not accomplished by the traditional functions of personnel administration. The most important work objective in the New American Hospital is not to serve patients but to *grow human resources*, for that is the only way the organization will be able to achieve its mission of service. People are resources just as much as money, physical plant, and technology. But unlike physical assets that *depreciate* in value over time, human resources have the unique capacity to grow, to *appreciate*! People can become more skilled, knowledgeable, committed, and courteous. The smart hospital is the one that finds ways to increase the return on the human assets it manages.

Existing personnel practices within the industry do not have this focus. They are oriented to an outdated industrial model that was primarily concerned with administering benefits and salaries, keeping records, and processing replaceable bodies through its selection system. This focus created a mechanical view of people that is chilling. The requirements of old-line personnel administration — that people are to do it by the numbers, stay behind the white line, and follow innumerable policies—do not accommodate the "ornery" independence of real people. The thinking went along this line: Do what's in your job description (don't do anything else), get in line with the organizational chart (so the chains of command will shackle you), and receive orderly step increases (forget the fact that some people are worth more and some are worthless!). It's equally instructive to think about what personnel departments in old-style hospitals do *not* do very well or at all—such functions as management development, team building, organizational renewal, wide-scale participative decision making in open ca- reer systems, delegation down the line, and promoting from within.

The New American Hospital pursues an approach that goes on a people offense. How can we get the most from our folks? How do we increase their skills and set their hearts on fire? Executives wishing to lead the revolution need to see the old personnel administration model as an enemy of their change agenda. Many of these practices have to be cleared away in a major philosophical repositioning of the department's function. Don't accept the limits of policy. Don't accept limits on your people's performance. Everything depends on the people.

Stop the Clock!

One symbolic way to begin is by doing away with the time clock. This symbol can be used to rapidly communicate to Associates the change in thinking and values that will be applied to them. The time clock is a mechanical way of collecting information about hours worked that makes the person an extension of a machine. It represents the assembly line reaching out to grab Associates as they walk in the door and is the last thing to let go of them as they leave for the day.

The message sent by taking Associates off the time clock and putting them on time cards is one of trust. Rather than seeing them as children who must be monitored, we trust them with time records just as we trust them with patients. Always make organizational change a symbolic act, one that is talked about and teaches values in such a way as to evoke head-nodding response from Associates.

One inspired hospital leader called as many Associates as could be spared out into the parking lot where a construction derrick was positioned. On his command, the time clock, which had been removed from the wall, was hoisted in the air. Then, in a voice tinged with emotion and personal commitment, he said, "Let this be clearly understood. You are not extensions of a machine, you are not the kind of people who would cheat this organization, and I refuse to let you be treated in this childlike manner. Henceforth you will complete your own time record because I trust you with time just as I trust you with our patients' lives. In this organization, people will be treated as adults. To do any less than that would be to disrespect who you are and I will not tolerate that."

At his signal, the crane operator dropped the time clock on the pavement. It gave a delicious clang! Amid cheers, the CEO strode away, leaving a group of dumbfounded Associates behind. Quicker than you can say, "You don't have to write a memo to explain things," the story went through the system — another brick added to the wall of excellence. The smashed time clock remains on display, a shrine where Associates bring their family members to see what once was.

Zapping Dead Programs

Recognizing an Associate of the Month is a good idea, as far as it goes. People of merit ought to be recognized in the organization. But Employee of the Month programs have become lifeless in their impact. Other programs such as Associate orientation are sometimes a waste of time. When the retirement plan is explained in great detail to eighteen-year-olds on their first day of employment, somebody just isn't thinking. When house publications print only noncontroversial topics, like a state-controlled press, one questions why management permits these things to go on.

Often these programs can be revitalized. In one New American Hospital, the Employee of the Month was renamed

Hero of the Month. Rewards were substantially increased, including getting the president's parking spot! Selection processes were upgraded so that those selected were truly exemplary.

Revitalization of old programs may work, but if the primary purpose is to teach or honor people, it may be necessary to create a whole host of programs, perhaps including some that operate for as few as three to six months, that are then replaced as a way to keep interest high and a sense of freshness in the organization. When it comes to people, don't support programs that go nowhere, do nothing, and aren't worth the time.

Rethinking the Personnel Department

A new mission for change must energize and reform the staff functions of the old personnel department and dramatically alter their influence throughout the organization. One way to start might be to rename it the People Division! Hospitals *are* a people business, and true reengineering of hospital management will require an expanded role for this function. Empowerment of the people certainly should also mean empowerment of this department.

Changing Policies to Support Managers. In our experience, every case of organizational renewal has required a complete review of existing personnel policy and practices. These policies are always too ponderous and interfering for the people they purport to serve; universally, managers complain about the negative impact they have on their people and on getting work done.

Equally damning is the negative effect personnel practices have on organizational change. Their overhaul should occur early in the change effort. If not, managers find frustration at every turn, unable to remove problem people, facing reward systems that reward only mediocrity, and forced to hire "warm bodies." Pay heed to the centurions of change when they request alteration of these practices.

Changing Personnel Executives to Support Line Managers. Because of the critical need for a radically new approach to leadership, it's imperative for the human resources executive to be a real heavyweight. Unfortunately, many hospital executives report that lightweight personnel administrators are prevalent in the industry. These managers were selected to run the old personnel administration functions, and their philosophy and departmental practices are often limited in scope. In some cases, the department manager has the desire and ability to retool the department quickly. The problem comes when the person in charge of personnel does not have the ability to make the change. There simply isn't time to retool these individuals in an organization undergoing rapid change. On the other hand, a great person in this job is a blessing for the change effort.

Some New American Hospital presidents have sent their human resources executives to Walt Disney University's course on people management, or to courses that outline excellent American and Japanese company people practices. Open up their thinking beyond the rigid look-alike models that we see in the hospital industry. Make whatever changes are necessary early on in order to reap an early harvest of returns from a renewed specialty. If you are replacing the human resources executive, I generally advise getting someone from outside the hospital industry who is up to speed with newer forms of people management.

The End of Demeaning Employeeism

Employeeism is a mindset that defines people as economic units of cost, thereby dehumanizing and demotivating them. The New American Hospital sees people for their possibilities and moves quickly to change the person-job equation.

Retooling Jobs for Dignity

When we refer to "lower levels" or people "up there," we impose a set of psychological perceptions based on a person's hierarchical positioning. This isn't conducive to building a society in which men and women can make their full contribution.

When a manager speaks of "my people," it sounds reminiscent of plantation slaveholders. Are they really "his people"? To say that people work for you is very different from saying that they work *with* you.

Language needs to be made more precise in American hospital management. Language is subtle. The women's movement showed how gender-gap language was detrimental to work achievement and career success for women. Earlier, minorities pointed out that using terms such as "boy" was a way in which to control African Americans. Similar to racism and sexism, employeeism is a way of keeping people in their place by using language that demeans them. In the long run, these practices and labels do as much damage to the employer as they do to the Associate.

Immediately stop using pejorative terms like "employee, subordinate, lower levels, and workers." Use language toward people that shows your sensitivity and courtesy.

Changing Associate Titles to Increase Role and Respect

Changing a person's name or title is an ancient technique signaling a change of roles and relationships. Abram was just a shepherd, but when his name was changed to Abraham, he became the father of many nations. Saul was a tentmaker on the road to Damascus with orders to kill Christians. When his CEO gave him a new commission, he became Paul! Ancient societies often rename young men as they enter manhood. In our own society, the common practice of a woman taking her husband's name also signals a change of relationship. What we call people affects how they think of themselves, and if we want them to think differently about themselves and their role within the organization, change names and titles.

At Decatur (Illinois) Memorial Hospital, Don Gent, the CEO, found old, demeaning names being used in the job classification system: Worker 1, Worker 2, Worker 3, Clerk 1, Clerk 2, Clerk 3. Picture yourself as a Clerk 2 at a neighborhood barbecue. When people ask what you do, do you say with pride, "I'm a Clerk 2"? Don quickly changed the titles, letting the job hold-ers have a major say in the project. It had a profound effect, yet it cost nothing to do.

Some people argue that upgrading titles is foolish, that calling a garbage collector a sanitary engineer is simply puffery. But suppose that your job was to pick up other people's trash, day in and day out, for thirty years. Would you want to be called a garbage collector, or would you rather have a different label? It takes very little to feel better about ourselves, and sometimes it takes little to make us feel small. Systematically eradicate labels that have no motivational content or that demean people. Which titles should we let people use? Ask them!

While you're at it, capitalize the word *Associate* wherever it appears in print, a no-cost way to demonstrate a deeper sym-bolism. Explain why you're doing it. Tie the change to the values statement, stating that it's a small but concrete way to express our respect for each other.

"R.E.S.P.E.C.T."

One of the top ten rock-and-roll songs of all time is Aretha Franklin's recording of "Respect." In the film *Brubaker*, Robert Redford plays a warden who walks in on a convict who is holding a knife at a guard's throat ready to take his life. Brubaker asks the question, "What do you want?" Filled with fear and rage, the convict gives voice to all his pent-up frustration by repeating Aretha's phrase, "R.E.S.P.E.C.T."

Respect is the one basic requirement we have for all our human interactions. You don't have to like me, you don't have to want me as your friend, but you must show me respect. Rodney Dangerfield says, "I don't get no respect." We've all been there. Courtesy and manners are the social expressions of mutual respect. Respect for yourself and respect from others are major components of your sense of self. In Oriental thinking, people lose face, or pride, when they act in a way that others do not respect.

What are we to make of the emotional and verbal abuse and profane language used by a few physicians on hospital staff?

When does a person's mistake at work ever justify being yelled at? What are we to make of a hospital supervisor who says to people, "If you don't want to do it my way we'll replace you with somebody who will." Are physicians so powerful or supervisors so elite that their priorities and need to vent are allowed precedence over the personal integrity of others? Move quickly to end any abusive interactions or lack of respect seen in the organization. Put it forever off-limits.

Staff abuse can only be ended by living the values of the organization. Some New American Hospitals have adopted policies that subject a violator who abuses an Associate to immediate loss of privileges or other penalties. This provides the political backing and ammunition the executive may need for enforcement. However, sometimes a physician has a bad day because the organization gave her a bad day. They didn't provide this Customer with the tools or supplies she needed in the way she needed them. An organization's failure to perform does not give the physician the right to spout off, but does justify her feeling frustrated. Therefore, the policy should specify that anytime the organization fails to respond, a task force will be convened within twenty-four hours to investigate and find a way to prevent the problem from recurring. Quick and timely response to organizational malfunction is promised. In exchange for that quick response, the physician is asked to preserve the team by bringing complaints to the appropriate party. Neither operating problems nor human disrespect are acceptable. Organizational change often hinges on powerful and symbolic tests such as this. Don't view it as a dreaded event — it's a way to underscore the value of the change program.

Learning to live with each other in a better way is not always easy, but it is always worth the price. What we want to do is create a renewed and powerful organizational culture, and Associates will be looking to see if management can pass the test. If we live the values, they are real. Unless leaders of change are willing to enforce them, values-centered management becomes meaningless and renewal momentum and credibility will be lost.

Back to Team Basics

Building a team isn't a matter of improving interpersonal functioning or a touchy-feely approach. The New American Hospital knows that getting a group of people to work together requires focusing on the fundamentals, the building blocks of team success.

Picking Winners by Tight Selection

Careless selection practices typify too many hospitals. The shortage of key technical and professional manpower has led to the practice of hiring "warm bodies." Marginal, mediocre, and sometimes malevolent employees are hired as the organization lets down its employment screens. If people have a license and are breathing, the thinking goes, they're good enough to work here.

The excellent organization knows that it can never be any better than its people — indeed, the organization is nothing but its people. Thus, there is a need to tighten up Associate selection processes so that the strongest, brightest, and best become members of the family. These people walk in the door with a different set of attitudes, a different level of pride, and a different commitment to personal performance. It's possible for a good manager to improve the levels of such qualities in people, but it's infinitely easier with people who have already learned some of these lessons in life.

A number of hospitals have begun using tighter selection procedures. While this takes more work than a twenty-minute interview, it's less work and trouble than trying to manage a problem case later on. These elements dramatically improve selection validity; it's more likely that you will pick a winner than a loser by following these procedures and systems:[2]

- Multiple interviewers and interviews
- Interviews of at least an hour in length

- Use of unusual interviewers such as those outside the technical area
- Use of retention profiles to spot those who are likely to stay on the payroll
- A short period of work sampling before the final hire

You can't win with losers. The first law of management is *selection*. Get that right and everything else you're going to do is easy. Get it wrong and everything else is *correction!*

Increasing the Investment in Training

Training is one of the surest ways management can signal: "We believe in your capacity for growth and ability to do more than we're asking." For all their technical expertise, hospital workers are often less trained than factory workers in other industries. In 1990 the average expenditure for training hospital Associates was $250. Compare that to the 1990 IBM expenditure of $2,200 per Associate. They made eleven times the bet that they could grow their people and stretch their ability to produce for the organization. The board of Motorola recently increased expenditures for Associate development from 2.8 percent to 3.5 percent of the expense budget. At Motorola, Associate development is seen as a strategic issue. Isn't it equally strategic to the business interests of a hospital?

Another way to think of the commitment to the development of human resources is to look at the amount of time budgeted for training and development. Hewlett-Packard Company has established a standard of 5 percent of working hours for all its divisions. That works out to two hours a week, or a hundred hours a year. If all hospital Associates were to receive two and a half weeks of Associate development annually, they would be on the same competitive fast track as Hewlett-Packard, a company in an extremely competitive industry that continues to post record sales, profitability, and gains in market share. They win because their people have the "smarts."

It's been said that Japan has the most educated bottom 50 percent of the work force anywhere in the world. That's a tremendous way to describe what an organization has to do to win. Associate development is a gamble, a bet made by management in a high-stakes poker game. The bet: If we invest in our people's skills to do their technical job and serve Customers, we will become more razorlike in our organizational performance. In the New American Hospital, we know we're in a lifetime learning situation as far into the future as we can see.

Increasing Retention by Assessing Turnover Causes

Organizations that win have lower turnover than their losing competitors, yet hospitals are typified by higher turnover rates than most other industries. *Turnover is the key measure of the human resource climate.* People simply do not stay in bad working situations. When an organization thinks it has a wonderful working environment, but people can hardly wait to leave, somebody doesn't have the facts straight. Inattention to turnover is a recipe for disaster, and it's a major symptom of hospitals that mismanage their people.

It's impossible to achieve organizational excellence when Associates are migrating in and out of an organization like so many nomads drifting across the desert sands. The retention of good Associates allows an organization to reap a harvest of talent and experience that takes years to acquire. Indeed, a key test of any organization is the degree to which it can hang onto good people. Most organizations have the ability to hire good people, but can they keep them?

Causes of turnover break down into two major categories. One is legitimate and justifiable, as when an Associate returns to school or moves out of state to accompany a spouse's career move; this accounts for one- to two-thirds of total turnover. The second category of turnover is unjustifiable — and possibly manageable. It includes Associates who leave to get a job elsewhere because of poor working relationships, lack of training, or limited career progress. It also accounts for one- to two-thirds of total turnover. Correcting some portion of this second category reduces the outflow of people that the organization has worked hard to find and has spent a lot of time, money, and effort orienting and bringing up to speed.

Every time we lose staff, it's like a brain losing some of its gray cells. After a while, the organization acts like it has Alzheimer's! Aggressively approach the retention problem by calculating a turnover budget. Multiply the number of turnovers by an estimated replacement cost, in order to calculate the amount of money that might be budgeted for retention strategies at no increase in cost to the organization. If a hospital employs 1,000 Associates and has a turnover rate of 10 percent, its loss of 100 Associates, multiplied by an estimated conservative replacement cost of $6,500 per head, costs $650,000 per year just for replacements.

The replacement cost includes separation payments, lost productivity while being short-staffed, increased overtime payments made to Associates during the departed Associates' absence, and costs of recruiting and moving replacements. Depending on how management compiles these costs, the replacement cost could be even higher than in the example above. If turnover could be cut 25 percent, then $162,500 could be used as a figure to fund projects associated with improving conditions that create turnover.

An organization that is losing good people cannot help but create an organizational climate of temporary and transitory affiliation. The New American Hospital sees people as members of the family, members we want to protect and keep. Stop the talent drain and create a great place to work. When Mt. Carmel Medical Center, Columbus, Ohio, began their change effort there were fifty registered nurse vacancies. They created an even more positive work setting, and two years later there was a waiting list of nurses wanting to get in. Imagine having so few vacancies that the personnel people have to work on other projects!

Monitoring Progress by Rerunning Opinion Surveys

Conducting an opinion survey of Associates is recommended shortly before or right after an organization's renewal effort

begins. Establish a baseline and identify blockages and problems affecting the staff. The survey should be rerun after twelve
to twenty-four months to determine which categories and question items have improved and which remain problems. These
data should be widely shared and heavily publicized to Associates to show them that the change effort is paying off for the
people as well as for the business. This is powerful information
and makes believers out of the cynical.

In 1986 Floyd Memorial Hospital, in New Albany, Indiana, ran its first opinion survey under its new president, John
White. There had been a publicly embarrassing series of revela-
tions about poor management, and morale was low. The hospital, a former county hospital operating on the outskirts of
Louisville against half a dozen stronger community hospitals,
was very poor in resources. The opinion survey documented
morale rates much lower than national norms. Eighteen months
later, in June 1988, the survey was conducted again (Figure 3.1).
In the interim there had been a tremendous organizational
renewal effort following the New American Hospital model. The
results show how much gain is possible in a short time frame
with good management concepts. The third round of surveying
in 1990 showed even greater gains.

Job Restructuring and the End of Pigeonholing

The problem with job descriptions is that they tell people what
they can't do. The minute we write on two pages of paper what
somebody can do, we've also just said not to do anything else!
Obviously, we don't want people running off and doing just
anything. We can't have housekeeping staff administering medi-
cations. But why do we want to make people fit job descriptions?
Why don't we fit jobs around what people can do?

I've often asked nurses why aides (an old hospital pejorative title) aren't allowed to do certain tasks. The answer I get
is, "They aren't trained." "But if aides don't do it, doesn't that
mean a registered nurse has to do it?" "Yes." "Well, if aides did it,
wouldn't that free you up to do other, more important tasks?"
"Yes, but aides aren't trained to do it." Restraining myself from

Figure 3.1. Opinion Survey Categories Compared After Renewal.

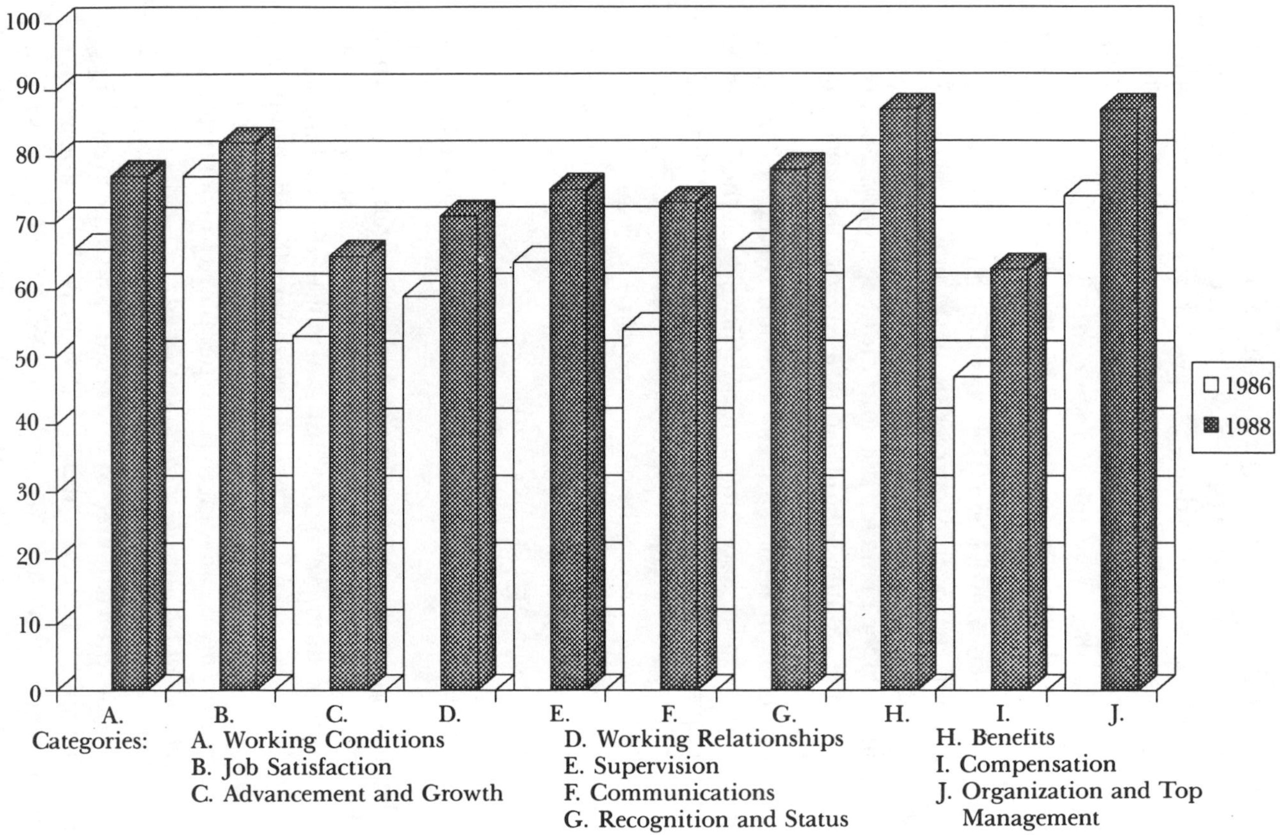

100
90
80
70
60
50
40
30
20
10
0
A.
B.
C.
D.
E.
F.
G.
H.
I.
J.
1986
1988
Categories:
A. Working Conditions
B. Job Satisfaction
C. Advancement and Growth
D. Working Relationships
E. Supervision
F. Communications
G. Recognition and Status
H. Benefits
I. Compensation
J. Organization and Top Management

taking a chair and bopping them, I ask, "Well, why don't you train them to do it?" Then comes the ultimate answer, which cannot be challenged because it is holy writ: "Well, it's not in their job description."

Contrast this approach with that of Panasonic, which follows their founder's advice, Matsushita's law, "If you see a problem around you, fix it." Panasonic, with 185,000 Associates worldwide, has no job descriptions. Matsushita's law is literally everybody's job description. If I see a problem but cannot fix it, my responsibility is to report what I see to someone who can.

I don't believe that hospitals are ready to eliminate job descriptions, but the reality strongly suggests making them more flexible and open. A general approach taken in the New American Hospital is consolidation and widening of job descriptions. Asking the fundamental questions of what people can do or can be trained to do makes it clear that we've cut the work pie into too many narrow slices. For example, cross-training and job rotation are possible, along with the possibility of collapsing several jobs into one.

Real People, Artificial Job Requirements

Many job descriptions and promotional channels are based on artificial job requirements such as degrees, length of service, or specialized experience. Where job requirements are mandated by state law or professional certification, the organization may have no choice but to comply. Where they are not required, consideration should be given to maximizing the use of people. *What counts is knowledge and experience, however it is acquired.* We need to stop thinking that people aren't capable and start thinking, "Why not give them a try!"

Job descriptions are an outgrowth of the assembly-line mentality of the early twentieth century. Jobs were broken down into the number of tasks a person could realistically perform in the assembly of a product within a short time span. Previously, in craft or farm jobs, people did a whole range of tasks and skills. Due to the tremendous latitude of these jobs, they seldom felt bored. There was so little repetition, so much variety, and so much freedom as to when work could be done that it used a person's full range of capabilities. Machine-age jobs changed all this. As jobs became smaller and smaller in content, the people doing them also found that they had less and less ability to learn other tasks, and after a period of time both management and Associates felt as if they were unable to do other things. But that's not reality. People can learn to do other jobs, and there isn't any reason why they shouldn't.

Riverside Hospital in Toledo, Ohio, saw the connection between Customer complaints of too many people parading in and out of their room and the need for people to have a greater sense of job identity and importance. Hospital managers asked, "Why don't we cross-train our people so that they can each do the other person's jobs?" They tried it and found that their staff were very interested and motivated. In time, this idea evolved into the creation of a single job description: "Patient Service Representative" (PSR). PSRs handled all of the housekeeping, meal delivery, visitor questions, and nurse assistant tasks. They were assigned individually to a block of patients on a particular floor to handle all of these needs. Each PSR now had a much larger job. They took personal responsibility for "their patients" and morale increased. Not surprisingly, turnover decreased. Customers were happier, and nursing managers were pleased to have someone in their unit to handle these tasks, instead of having to call on several different departments. As a goal, try to reduce the number of job titles in your organization by 50 percent.

Misapplied Job Standards Stifle Job Performance

One of the newest gimmicks in hospital personnel administration is writing quantifiable job standards for all the tasks and functions performed on each job. For some reason this assembly-line mentality becomes more creative and intricate as it reaches the end of its serviceable lifetime! This project requires unbelievable worker-hours to accomplish. Why do we do this?

W. Edwards Deming observed that old industrial engineering approaches can be misused; they must be applied to group processes and work standards, not to individuals. Four decades later, the hospital industry has found a new dead-end to go down and is spending what little resources remain on an approach that produces nothing.

Better alternatives abound. Why not set up standards of performance for the work group, specifying the work that must be accomplished and the level at which it must be accomplished? Focusing on group standards, group performances, and systems that emphasize team behavior has always been found to be more effective than focusing on controlling individuals. When the emphasis is on what the group does, group norms tend to monitor or correct what individuals are doing. It takes less work and accomplishes a lot more.

Enriching Jobs for Achievement and Growth

Job descriptions tend to be a boring list of repetitive duties to which the job holder has been assigned. Later, management doesn't understand why the Associate says, "It's not my job." Management sets up the game and is then surprised when Associates follow the rules. A human resources approach might put a different spin on the normal static state of jobs by building a change segment into them. In hospitals where managers do quarterly work planning, it is easy to look at the list of new projects for pieces of work that can be delegated to Associates. Thus, a salad maker might be given a specific project to develop a new recipe or to write up suggestions for changing the work flow to make four hundred salads per shift.

Accomplishing a specific target brings a renewed sense of achievement. This may take the form of establishing a better standard of performance in the same job. A Marriott busboy who must deliver room service orders within a specified fifteen-minute delivery period has a greater sense of achievement than one who works elsewhere and delivers an order whenever he gets around to it. Placing requirements on people, and making the work fit into an achievement mode, is a test, and people like passing tests. They like proving themselves in the workplace.

Wherever this can be done — and creative managers usually have no trouble finding places where it can be done — it adds another element of zest, productivity, and pride.

Job Security, Downsizing, and Problem Employees

In an organization with a need to reduce its head count and still remain committed to excellence, it's imperative to get rid of problem people and keep good ones. A hospital that won't fire problem people puts the job security of good people at risk. Thinking of this as a group defensive posture puts a very different perspective on it. Start immediately to remove or rehabilitate people who do not perform up to the organization's standards or who violate values.

Most attorneys advise organizations to lay people off on the basis of seniority. But if a hospital management hasn't removed problem people earlier, this means that they will have to keep them and get rid of newer hires who are good performers! It also means problem people now represent a greater percentage of the remaining work force! Turnover studies show that good people tend to leave on their own accord, while poor performers hang on forever. The clear prescription: move first on problem workers before reducing the head count by layoffs. More than cutting the fat before cutting the lean, this is cutting out the cancer before cutting the lean.

Problem Managers or Problem Employees?

Typically we find that most hospitals accumulate problem employees whose performances are unacceptable. Studies have shown that about half of problem employee behaviors indicate problem supervision. When employees are not appropriately selected, orientation and job training programs are weak, leadership is lacking, standards of performance are poorly defined, and rewards are absent, it's not surprising that behavior goes off-track.

Just as laying off Associates is not the best solution to an organization's economic problems, so, too, a case can be made that the timing of corrective actions against problem employees might better follow the rehabilitation of the hospital's management team. A recharged and renewed manager who has a better understanding of his or her role may be able to more positively turn around problem behaviors.

Working to Produce Job Security

The New American Hospital works to provide steady and secure employment for its members. This means avoiding mass layoffs if they can be prevented. The IBM model is instructive at this point in that it is not the company's policy not to lay people off but has been a long-standing practice. No one can guarantee that a layoff will never come, but the intent to avoid layoffs should be both announced and practiced. However, holding job security inviolate does not apply to individual poor performers. No one has the right to expect a job to be safe if he or she does not do that job. And inviolate job security also does not mean that we may never have to reduce the size of our work force.

Layoffs Aren't Creative

The management that can't come up with any answers for its problems other than laying people off just isn't thinking. Nothing is as deadly as a layoff. It creates widespread anxiety and insecurity, adds to the work pressures of the remaining staff, causes a deterioration in the worth of management, proves the organization incapable of meeting security needs, and creates union risks. It is a gross violation of the unwritten contract between labor and management; any management that resorts to this answer can be considered to be failing. Layoffs represent the grossest misunderstanding of how human organizations function, by destroying the organization's human spirit and soul to save a few dollars. For years hospitals trumpeted that they were caring places, centered on human values, but the first time they encountered business difficulties they were willing to be uncaring and sacrifice people. When the accountants run your business, all is lost.

If any discussions are currently being held in your organization about layoffs, stop them. If there have been layoffs in the past, make a vow not to let any more occur. There are other ways to meet downsizing needs. People are not simply economic units of cost. The New American Hospital searches for more creative cost solutions than the destruction of Associates' job lives and the unhappiness of their families.

The true problem that leads to layoffs is a need for cost reduction. Instead of laying people off, create pressure to find creative ways of reducing costs and increasing revenue. It isn't always easy to do this, and some hospitals have lost their opportunity. At the very least, let Associates see management struggling to save jobs. Remember that if layoffs do become necessary, there will be negative morale effects for years, recruitment will be harder, and trust will be more difficult to recapture.

Following the Rules of Head-Count Reduction

First, preserve the human environment in which the organization does its work. Hospitals cannot afford the mass disruptions caused by layoffs. Ask yourself: Has everything been done short of a layoff to reduce costs and waste? Is there anything we can do to increase revenues? Have we truly been creative in finding other options?

Second, enlist Associates' cooperation in reducing costs or increasing revenues. Provide full disclosure of the organization's economic difficulties. Share any relevant financial data. Say to people, "We're intending to live up to our practice of providing job security, but we need your help because we must find new ways to do things, new ways to be more productive, new ways to cut costs, and new ways to increase revenue." Use brainstorming sessions, ideation channels, and creation of task forces to start piecing together a solution. Establish a deadline when these numbers must be met.

Third, handle head-count reduction by attrition, early retirement, retraining, and redesigning jobs. Attrition is easier to achieve in large departments such as nursing than in smaller departments where positions can't be left open. Communicate clearly that it may be necessary for Associates to learn new jobs or transfer to other departments.

And fourth, vow never to do this again. If old ways of thinking hadn't prevailed for so long, you wouldn't have been caught in this bind. Do it right the first time, and realize that every piece of bad management comes out of some-body's hide.

Notes

1. Harvard Business School Case Services, *The Lincoln Electric Company* (Boston, Mass.: Harvard Business School, 1975), p. 7.
2. V. Clayton Sherman, *From Losers to Winners: How to Manage Problem Employees, and What to Do if You Can't* (New York: AMACOM, 1987), pp. 37 ff.

4

Delivering the Service Strategy

Institutions that can no longer provide their customers with a
product they want to buy at a price they want to pay for it have
lost the right to survive. This is a harsh judgment. It is the
judgment of the marketplace and of the customers for whom
we all compete.

— Edward R. Telling
Chairman emeritus,
Sears, Roebuck & Co.
(Last successful Sears leader
before the Wal-Mart onslaught)

The only reason for any organization to exist is to serve its
Customers. While hospitals perform admirably, even mirac-
ulously, in serving most Customers, it has become clear that
there are gaps in service, omissions in relationships and attitudes, and lower levels of patient satisfaction than are desirable. Many hospitals are innovating, and much experimenting is
going on. This chapter proposes to pull together all of the many
good ideas into a comprehensive strategy, pulling out all the
stops and covering all the bases that would improve Customer
service. That strategy has three major parts: first, dealing with
Customer communications in a way that reduces the confusion
they experience; second, making the system respond to improve
the delivery of care as Customers experience it; and finally,
setting high standards of performance and measuring the organization against them.

Designing a Comprehensive Service Strategy

In working to create fully functioning hospitals, I have continually been struck with the unacceptably high degree of dissatisfaction that exists among too many hospital Customers. To

respond to that dissatisfaction, many hospitals began in the 1980s to institute new approaches to Customer service. For example, Steve Ummel, CEO of Memorial Hospital, South Bend, Indiana, during the mid 1980s used the Marriott Corporation and the Hyatt Corporation as benchmark companies in designing a Customer service strategy. This kind of innovative thinking and search for better approaches is now going on in a wide range of hospitals. The general management literature on Customer service has also been expanding, and a number of excellent sources are now available (see the Recommended Readings in the back of this book). How can we best use this exploding knowledge as part of reinventing the hospital?

My purpose is to propose that all these ideas be pulled together into a comprehensive strategy. Some hospitals have developed training in guest relations, while others have pursued more sophisticated techniques such as Customer measurement, added services, physician account management, or guaranteed service levels. Rather than pursuing a few of these approaches on a piecemeal basis, we can bring them all together under the roof of the New American Hospital. This chapter will attempt to lay out the range of elements that might be included in a total strategy, where the synergy of the individual parts becomes greater than the sum of the parts.

The individual elements of the Customer service strategy that follow are grouped into the following categories: Customer communication, making service systems work, and setting standards and measuring results:

- *Customer communication* includes strategies for building an open flow of communication to and from the Customer, visitors, and physicians. Not a public relations campaign, the communication strategy recommends open communication to help Customers and visitors access services. This means listening to complaints and solving problems immediately. Seek out Customers' expectations, and then meet and exceed them.

- *Making the system respond* includes strategies for opening up the organization to change, removing irritations, adding value to present services, and obtaining Associates' participation and support. It is in this area that literally hundreds of changes will be made during the organization's renewal.

• *Setting standards and measuring results* includes specifying high standards, devising ways to measure how well the organization has done in the Customer's eyes, and being concerned with measurement more as a change tool than as an academic study.

Who Is the Customer?

"The Customer is King," wrote Marshall Field. "The Customer is always right," wrote John Wanamaker. Serving the Customer is the end objective of all management activity. As one hospital CEO said recently, "The choice is clear. Either serve the Customer, serve those that are serving the Customer, or get out." This is tough and demanding language, yet it shows clear thinking that is markedly absent in too many hospitals. Many organizations clearly do not value their Customer; then their executives wonder why they are beset with competitive problems and shrinking market share. The Customer is our partner, not an annoyance or simply a cash box.

The usual definition of the Customer is the bill-paying person at the end of an organization's product-service delivery pipeline. The problem with such a limited definition is that most people in organizations have little or no direct interaction with that Customer. As a result, the service orientation is lost, and departments begin to focus on turf, procedural controls, internal problems, and a host of lesser issues. This organizational drift eventually results in rigid, nonserving entities whose original purpose becomes forgotten.

Whoever is the beneficiary of your talent and effort is your Customer. This broader definition means that staff units view line units as their Customers, not simply as higher-status or higher-power groups. It also means that executives truly work *for* their Associates. It is they who are in closer proximity to the king.

This definition also means that there are many Customer

groups. It is foolish to argue whether the doctor or the patient or some other group is our Customer; instead, we must get on with meeting the needs of these folks. All the Customer groups must be served. Sometimes these groups have conflicting priorities — life isn't easy — but there is less risk in overserving than in underserving. The hospital's Customers include patients and physicians, families and visitors, other departments and Associates, the community, employers, and vendors. It is difficult to serve all these Customer groups and balance the priorities, but it is better to overserve than to accept the risk of underserving.

New American Hospitals have launched a thorough search to find ways to serve the king better. Yet the winning hospital also knows that there are limitations in its ability to be of service. Every business chooses its Customers in terms of the kinds of products and services that it provides. No business can be all things to all people, and so a basic question arises that every organization must answer: What Customers can we serve, and what are the limits to what we can offer them?

Managing Service Basics

Customers often report high levels of dissatisfaction with the hospital services they receive. But not for long. Unhappy Customers tend to go elsewhere to have their needs met. Customer-satisfaction levels are the difference between business growth and business failure. The following basic principles can help guide the formation of a service strategy.

Treat Your Customers as Lifetime Partners. Ask Customers continuously the two most important questions: How are we doing? and How can we make it better? By establishing communication mechanisms and systems to find out what Customers want, we obtain a continual stream of needed information about their expectations.

Look at Your Business Through the Customers' Eyes. Wise executives make it their practice to see, hear, smell, taste, and feel what their Customers experience during any contact with the business. One executive checked himself into his hospital's emergency room and asked the staff to treat him as if he had been brought in with a broken leg. He wanted to see the hospital from the Customers' perspective — lying down.

Deliver More Than You Promise. Perceived service is the difference between what Customers expect and what they get. Make sure that every service or product you provide for your Customers does all you said it would do — and then some. Your willingness to go the extra mile will set you apart from the also-rans who perceive Customers' expectations as the maximum required instead of a starting platform for exceptional service. Bill Gonzalez, CEO of Butterworth Hospital, Grand Rapids, Michigan, speaks of "Astonishing service. Miracle service. Incredible service." He backs up this rhetoric with high organizational standards in terms of Customer ratings of the hospital's performance. Says Gonzalez, "If the Customer isn't happy, nobody's happy!"

Focus Everyone's Efforts on Rewarding the Customer. Ask Associates to answer this question: What results do we produce, and how do they benefit the Customer? Then ask each person or group to set specific measurable service improvement goals, complete with deadlines. Involving Associates through Customer satisfaction teams (CSTs) and other approaches makes Customer service *the* top priority.

Select and Train Associates in the Art of Quality Customer Service. An effective training program makes the organization's service goals clear and attainable, conveying information about products, services, and benefits. Focus problem-solving ideas on identifying and managing "moments of truth — every occasion of Customer contact.

Reward Everyone for Rewarding the Customer. People do what is rewarded. Create a workable system that gives rewards to Associates who provide great service. Rewarding the Customer is everyone's job, but rewarding those who reward the Customer is management's job. Properly carried out, it becomes a triple reward system, because the Customer, organization, and Associate all win. Start recognizing outstanding service immediately!

Capitalize **Customer** *in All Publications and Correspondence.* Capitalizing *Customer* wherever it appears in print is a no-cost approach to signaling the importance of this group, and their centrality to our mission. Some would argue that it isn't correct grammatical style, but it's good management, and Customers won't object!

Copy Successful Customer Service Practices in Benchmark Companies. The desire to serve Customers is not new in the hospital industry, but the fanaticism to do it at extremely high levels is. One way to cut learning time is to dispatch various departmental personnel to excellent service companies outside the industry.

Executive Coordination of Customer Strategy

The job of setting up a coordinated service strategy is beyond the scope of the marketing department alone and should be done by an interdisciplinary management team. Our experience suggests the value of having the CEO or COO be at least an ex officio member of this steering committee and of assigning a high priority to executive monitoring of its progress. Each of the major areas described in this chapter is assigned to a task force that in turn may divide the problem up among numerous Do It Groups (DIGs), or project teams. The group responsible for coordination of the Customer service strategy should evaluate different projects in terms of their urgency, importance, ease of implementation, and other relevant criteria. This can be used to identify which projects should be tackled immediately.

From the strategy group, through the task forces, a tactical plan is created that aggressively attacks the problem. St. Mary's Medical Center in Evansville, Indiana, completed a tactical plan in sixty days that identified over two hundred projects, established priorities, and set quarterly assignments so that all of the projects could be completed in the following twelve months.

The executive's primary task is to see that a tactical work plan is evolved for implementing the Customer service strategy. Work groups will be making recommendations on each of the items in the plan. Some of these groups may become stalled or make shortsighted recommendations. Don't expect the individual work groups to drive this important part of the organizational change effort. Executives must drive strategy in order to get results as rapidly as possible; results then provide change energy, which reinforces the message that the renewal effort is on-track and worth the work.

Outstanding Customer service is the result of a dedicated, coordinated strategy by the organization. Executive responsibility includes developing and implementing the strategy, getting acceptance for it by Associates and managers, establishing service expectations, eliminating duplicate efforts and recognizing outstanding service results.

Keeping an Eye on the Market. Dealing well with Customers through excellent service is the backbone of the hospital's overall marketing strategy. Nothing succeeds like success, and nothing will spread faster than positive word of mouth in the community. But as important as "Wow" service is, it is not sufficient to deal with some of the wider marketing questions that should be addressed.

Studies of competitive strategy have shown convincingly that an organization needs to position itself wisely in the market. A hospital that doesn't position itself as having either the best quality, the lowest price, or some specialty or unique service not obtainable elsewhere will be vulnerable to attack. Add to this market reality the economic pinch of the current reimbursement system, and there is a convincing argument to be made that hospitals must carefully avoid the service extension trap. Pick service and product lines carefully; then provide excellent service and success will be yours.

The wise hospital executive makes the organization a market winner as a way to set a tone of achievement. Associates like to hear and read that the organization is winning and doing new things. A misconception would be that when an organization is retooled into a New American Hospital, all its business problems are going to evaporate. The successful executive pursues other strategies in marketing, finance, collaboration, and joint ventures with physicians. If members of the organization see in press announcements that new marketing programs are being started they feel that the organizational spirit is healthy. The tone of achievement creates a winning momentum on which the smart executive can piggyback his or her organizational change program. Thus there is a dynamic synergy, an excitement, created by the process of the organization's marketing success and its renewal effort.

Targeting Serviceable Customer Groups. What can you do well? What shouldn't you do at all? Don't waste time trying to be what your competitor is, or what you shouldn't be. Unfortunately, we can't fill everybody's needs, so let's do a superb job filling those we can.

Identify market niches and stake out competitively defensible positions. To the extent possible, don't go toe-to-toe with your competitors or you'll run the risk of becoming a commodity provider. Instead pick out areas of specialization. When that's not possible, and when your competitors offer identical services, the only way to compete is to add value and outdo them in service.

Evaluating Departments on Service, Quality, and Price. It is around these three variables that organizations tend to win or lose in a competitive market. Value can be defined as quality received for the cost expended. Hospital Customers clearly are sending two messages: drive the quality up and drive the cost down. To truly be a Customer-serving organization, hospitals must respond to those two commands. New American Hospitals are learning that as quality is increased, costs decrease. Doing a systematic review of these questions in each department has always been helpful to sharpen the focus on what's being offered.

Discontinue outlived programs. The best way to succeed is to identify the market segments the organization can serve well and concentrate resources there. This important and simple concept must be followed in taking on new market exposure, but it must be applied with equal vigor to current services that have outlived their usefulness. Many organizations become involved in marginal efforts that are ego-satisfying, but that do nothing but eat cash.

Does the Organization Fit What the Customer Wants? If not, change it! Pursue the logic that the Customer may know more about the business of being a provider than you do. This may not be true about technical care functions, and there may be exceptions to the rule, but start with the idea that Customer complaints reveal misfitting points of interaction. All organizations are ultimately judged on the question of how well they fit Customers' wants and needs.

Effective Customer Communication

Effective managers collect Customer input and change the organization to fit. When an organization's managers do what they're told, Customers are able to teach them their business. If they listen well, all that's left to do is to follow the king's orders. Minnesota Mining and Manufacturing Company (3M) reports that more than 50 percent of their new product and service innovations come from following up on Customer complaints. "Listen, believe, and do," said Sam Walton of Wal-Mart Stores. Let the Customer teach you your business, then change the business.

Business 101 as Taught by the Customer

If the Customer is to be the teacher, channels for input must be established. Where and how can we learn the lessons?

1. *Give greater credence to reports.* Listen to reports from Nursing or other units that directly interact with the final Customer. What do these groups say is needed? Believe what they tell you and respond immediately.
2. *Spend time with the Customer.* At least once a week, every member of management should spend a minimum of half a day with Customers. Learn their problems, find out where the glitches are. If you want to be more organized about it, routinely hold focus groups to identify general problem areas or probe a particular problem in depth. Believe what Customers tell you and do it.
3. *Practice "naive listening."* Forget for a moment your expertise and what you think you know about your specialty. Listen naively to what your Customer is saying, as though you didn't know anything about the subject.
4. *Call yourself up.* Call your department and play the role of a Customer, or have someone do it for you. How well did your

group react? Call yourself again, and this time make it a more complicated problem, or be a little irritating. Now how well did your group do?

5. *Read and post every Customer complaint.* Let everyone in the department see it on the wall. Ask, "How can we fix this so it doesn't happen again?" Respond to each complaint within twenty-four hours. Post every compliment, too. Broadcast in every way possible that what you stand for is Customer service.

These mechanisms put the people who do the work into a direct feedback loop from their Customers. The staff's natural desire to want to meet Customer expectations will do the rest.

Reexamine Basic Information Packages

It is said, "You never get a second chance to make a first impression." Communicating information clearly to Customers makes them feel welcome and at ease. Conversely, poor signage tells Customers that finding their way easily is not as important to you as it is to them. The objective is to reduce Customers' frustration and disorientation by providing them with the information they need to find their way, access services, and feel more at ease. There are many ways to provide this information:

- *Hospital maps.* Patients and visitors are confused with the maze of hallways and departments that make up the modern health care complex. Maps that are available throughout the hospital can effectively convey this information. Signage and map information should be checked for consistency as well as accuracy. Other media may be helpful, or some form of electronic directory or custom printout of directions such as the one offered by the Hertz Corporation. Complementing these aids are Associates and auxilians—do *they* know their way around the facility?

- *Services directory.* Another needed piece is a services directory, indicating how Customers access services. Hotels provide effective services directories for their Customers; they are a benchmark source of ideas.

*   *Fire safety instructions.* Fire safety and fire exit instructions should be clear. Some hospitals do this on a continuous broadcast over closed-circuit television modeled after those of the leading hotel chains.
*   *Telephone card.* Another useful idea from the hotel industry is a telephone card listing common communication points within the hospital. This should prominently display the Customer Hot Line number.
*   *Instructions for patients and visitors.* A frequent friction point is what hospital visitors can and can't do. These rules were usually formulated to ensure the safety and comfort of all patients, but they sometimes create hurt feelings or a bad image. Visitor orientation instructions can prevent many problems. Associates in Customer contact areas such as Nursing or Admitting can identify what kinds of information requests are most frequent and should be included.

The key to each of these ideas is to provide your Customers with as much information as they need. It also increases staff productivity when Customers can tell you what they want with a minimum of effort. Once Customers are provided with this information, it is essential to *deliver* the service they deserve and exceed the expectations they had when they entered.

Making the System Respond

As Customers experience the delivery system, they see a number of things that irritate them as well as things that need to be added. Rather than dismissing their observations, the New American Hospital learns, then changes the system.

Removing Customer Irritations and Complaints

Consider these long-standing, nonresponsive Customer practices of the old hospital:

- Patients in pain and discomfort are required to wait for long periods in Admitting.
- Patients' sleep is disturbed by noisy carts, paging, or staff interruptions in the room.
- Visiting rules convenience the staff rather than serving the needs of the patient.

This lack of response to obvious need is carried out by concerned health service professionals who believe they know best. Another form of nonresponse is "smoothing feathers." Staff members are often put in the position of saying, "We're sorry," without being allowed, expected, or required to change the system. Complaint handling that doesn't change the system is the sorriest sort of nonresponse.

Improving Operations by Removing Complaints. Begin by listing all the complaint areas you know of. Get the staff involved. Include complaint letters and any survey results available, and ask Customers for suggestions. Identify the biggest or most essential problems and go to work to eliminate them. Following are some of the common problems often found in hospitals. Do any apply to your operation?

- Inability to keep to a work schedule
- Long waiting times
- Demeaning gown
- Lack of privacy
- Dirty waiting areas
- Impersonal staff attitude
- Nickel-and-dime charges for services such as television and parking
- Unattended patients left in hallways between services
- Poor signage
- Slow response to service and personal requests
- Excessive telephone transfers between departments
- Unnecessary restrictions on family members
- Unclear billing or multiple bills
- Long waits for equipment or tests

Some complaints may not be solvable. Perhaps the practice of a department's specialty requires some inconvenience for the Customer, or budget limitations may make it impossible to get rid of every annoyance. All the more reason to remove all the negatives you can, and to soften the impact of those you can't.

Resolving Complaints. A telephone Customer Hot Line and a "Give Us Your View" postcard evaluation are two useful tools for immediate resolution of complaints. However, they represent only a stopgap measure if the more positive elements of the Customer service strategy are not implemented. This portion of the strategy is designed to resolve complaints quickly in order to avoid Customer defections and subsequent negative publicity.

When resolution of complaints takes too long, Customer satisfaction drops substantially. One study found that 70 percent of customers would do business again with an organization that resolved a complaint in their favor, but 95 percent would do business with them again if the problem was resolved on the spot. Rapid resolution of complaints actually builds Customer loyalty. It is imperative that both the Hot Line and the "Give Us Your View" card system give authority to staff to resolve the problem directly with the Customer.

The ideal telephone Customer Hot Line includes around-the-clock staffing and a number for any Customer to call with either praise or complaint. This service is for use by Customers or visitors in nonmedical situations to report any problems regarding hospital service (cleanliness of room, food quality, etc.). If the caller lodges a Customer service complaint, the Hot Line follows up by contacting the appropriate party to provide immediate attention to the problem.

After an appropriate period of time—twenty or thirty minutes—the Customer Hot Line contacts the caller again to make sure that the problem was solved. If not, the Hot Line contacts the administrator-on-call for follow-up. Calls are tracked by category and quantified to reveal trouble spots. Do It Groups (described in Chapter Five) are started for problems that require them, or they're referred to the appropriate departmental Customer Satisfaction Team (discussed later in this chapter). This program is actively promoted by having the Hot Line number placed on all phones, and by providing information in communication vehicles such as the information guide, phone indexes, and closed-circuit TV.

One hospital had its managers field Hot Line calls in rotation; managers who did not meet housewide minimum service standards had to staff the Hot Line two or three times as often as their peers who were meeting the standard. In effect, this rewarded managers with excellent Customer service and increased the service awareness of managers who needed improvement!

The "Give Us Your View" postcard contains a short message from the CEO regarding the hospital's quest for excellence and the importance of Customer input. The card could ask a few open-ended questions such as:

- How could we have made your experience here better?
- In our effort to be excellent, what would you suggest we change?
- Let us know if any Associates showed [add values statement] during your visit so we can show our appreciation.
- Has anything good or bad happened during your visit that you want us to know about?

The card also asks if Customers want a personal response and, if so, how to contact them. The card is available throughout the hospital. Drop boxes are placed in numerous locations such as waiting rooms. If a problem needs immediate response, the card would direct the Customer to the Hot Line. Cards are collected at least daily, delivered to a designated executive's office for immediate resolution, and tabulated to identify recurring problems.

Adding Value to Services

The concept of adding value is that it is important to add to your services and products something extra that is not provided by your competitors. Ask what else you could do, *in each department,* that would add value and make what you do better and more appreciated by your Customers. *Caveat:* A possible trap of the value-added concept is going after shadow instead of substance, fluff instead of significant change.

If a hospital were designed physically and programmatically by its Customers, what would it look like? What kind of furniture would be in the rooms, what colors would the walls be painted, what size would rooms be, what kinds of interactions would occur between the staff and the Customer? The Marriott creates mock-ups of hotel rooms, then parades Customers through to get their reactions. Customers decide the shape of the rooms and their color scheme. Every organization needs to suspend its expertise and listen to Customers, and learn from what they have to say.

Monitor Service Enhancements and Performance. As successive changes are made in the organization's practices, procedures, and programs, it's important to monitor how they are performing as new offerings and to debug them as rapidly as possible. Further monitoring at this point depends on how well each of these new programs is doing. In the continual experimental laboratory that the organization represents, even Customer-directed changes can backfire and produce too little return for the organization.

Provide Meetings and Mechanisms for Problem Solving. For real problem solving, it is important to get decision makers together and set deadlines in order to push solutions rapidly through the system. Unfortunately, in many hospitals such mechanisms and response patterns are not part of the system. People say that they're short-staffed and too pressed with other priorities. These organizations inadvertently wind up defending the status quo rather than changing and developing the organization. Are processing mechanisms in place in your hospital, or is the organization so busy operating that it doesn't have time to get any work done?

Create Change in Existing Services. The progress of research and development at General Motors Corporation went awry in the 1980s when the corporation invested its financial and manpower resources into designing ultrasophisticated futuristic cars. The organization needed to stop spending R&D money on future cars and devote that effort into fixing problems in the existing product line. For the New American Hospital, it may make sense to consider fixing current service cycles before moving off into newer projects. Let's do things right before starting something new.

Be Prepared to Work on Small Suggestions. Don't be surprised to find out that Customers often ask for small improvements. Can a service be made easier to use? Could a sequence be changed? Could a product be packaged differently? Often large, complex technology and organizations are judged by small details. Attention to the small yields gigantic results. Don't make the mistake of dismissing as inconsequential the small items that Customers ask for.

Add Value to Present Products. Management's success is based on continually improving what is offered, not in serving the same stale program over and over. The product or service you're offering is not limited to what it is now. What else could it be? What could be added to make it fill another need? If you don't know the answer to these questions, ask your Customers — they can tell you.

Begin by listing all possible improvements. Get the staff involved. Include Customers' suggestions. Identify the biggest or most essential concepts that would improve what you do. Following are value-added ideas that have worked in some hospitals. Do any apply to your operation?

1. *General health care*
   - Home visits
   - Free flu shots
   - Free cholesterol or blood pressure screening
   - Free Medicare and Medicaid counseling
   - Preregistration
   - In-room admissions/registration
   - Outpatient housing
   - Post-treatment counseling
   - Trailer hookups
   - Transitional living facilities
   - Twenty-four-hour hospital information channel
   - Automated patient signout via television

2. *Transportation*
    *   Doorman or other assistance with luggage
    *   Valet parking
    *   Free local transportation
    *   Museum trips
    *   Vaccines and health service available to overseas travelers
    *   Security escort service to car after dark
3. *Children and families*
    *   Bedside accommodations for families
    *   Twenty-four-hour family visiting
    *   Automated family education concerning patient's condition
    *   Carnivals
    *   Children's parents allowed in operating rooms
    *   Children's videotape library
    *   College scholarships
    *   Community information about tourism, restaurants, churches
    *   Free clothing to patients or families in need
    *   Dormitories, apartments, low-cost or free housing, or guest houses for families
    *   Family suites
    *   Stuffed animal zoo
    *   Summer camp
    *   Parents allowed to "room in" with their children
    *   School tutoring
    *   Toy store
    *   Babysitting services
    *   Children's play area
    *   Day care
    *   Sick-child care
4. *Culinary services*
    *   Candlelight dinner for maternity patients
    *   Full-service restaurant
    *   Gourmet and kosher menus
    *   Kitchen facilities for visitor or patient use

- Food accessibility on floor, vending machines, and room service
- Expanded hours for food service availability
- Policy of allowing visitors to eat in patients' rooms
- Picnic basket at discharge

5. *Room services*
- Creature comfort, such as recliners in patients' rooms
- Better architectural design, more private rooms, or wards with movable walls
- Redesign of the nurses' station to make it geographically closer to patients, or to make it psychologically closer by removing fortresslike counters
- Lower cost of rooms if family provides some support services during stay

6. *Other*
- Arts-and-crafts supplies available
- Backrubs
- Library and in-hospital video store
- Fitness-exercise room
- Showers and laundry for visitors
- Multilingual staff or free interpreters
- Provisions for business meetings, including secretarial help
- VIP suites including videocassette recorder, refrigerator, and microwave

As part of organizational renewal, an assignment should be made for each manager to identify, implement, and report on all possible items that could be added by way of improvements or additions to services in their department.

Gaining Associates' Commitment

How do we get Associates ready, willing, and able to jump on the Customer service bandwagon? Unless they see something in it for them, this could be a failed strategy.

Remove Grievances and Irritations. Associates can focus on the team's objectives only when they aren't concerned with what the system is or isn't providing to meet their personal needs. Unhappy troops don't win the battle! Sometimes what is needed is an attitude survey of Associates to determine where the friction points are. This kind of study, done properly, is a powerful management tool for improving the climate of the organization as well as for increasing job satisfaction and productivity. But remember that once attitude research has been conducted, it is essential to act on the findings and respond to Associates' needs. If the problems are not resolved, dissatisfaction will only intensify.

Is Guest Relations Training Really Needed? Managers often ask, "Is guest relations training really necessary?" Is the answer to service problems a learning sequence of orientation, training, and reinforcement? Is the problem really that the staff don't know how to do their jobs or have a poor attitude? Or is the problem that their irritations are caused by system and operational problems that result in poor Customer service? Guest relations or "smile" training can be ineffective if the training does not actually minimize negative experiences with Associates on the firing line. Some organizations have found that by improving Customer-service systems, guest relations training becomes moot. My judgment is that I would use guest relations training to cap the foundational pieces of good Associate treatment. Why not make it an end strategy, rather than a beginning point for enhancing Customer service?

Walt Disney said, "Customer relations simply mirror employee relations." Treat people well and make the work environment so comfortable, exciting, and rewarding that people truly enjoy their jobs and working for their organization. Good Customer relations are a natural result of this process. American hospitals have too frequently followed a counterfeit approach. They lay people off, don't stand by them during economic downturns, allow the staff to be abused by a few physicians, provide insufficient training and job mobility, and create the kind of terrible work environment that leads inevitably to high turnover rates. And when Customer complaints rise, they send all these Associates to guest relations training. If you work in a bad environment, the guest relations message is perceived as saying, "Even though we're kicking you in the shins, smile." This cynicism simply doesn't work.

L. L. Bean's version of the Golden Rule was "Treat your employees the way you want them to treat your customers." By creating the kind of organization that Associates love to work for, L. L. Bean has very little turnover (for example, they pay their Associates 20 percent more than the industry average because they believe that the result is 40 percent more productivity). The kind of Customer service and courtesy for which L. L. Bean is world-famous is not a result of guest relations training, but of superior human treatment by management.

The Adopt-a-Patient Program. Under this approach each patient entering the hospital is assigned to an Associate or manager. This staff person is not primarily a personal "complaint Hot Line," but is a welcoming representative who provides a visible expression of concern for the Customer's satisfaction and comfort while at the hospital.

Everyone should be assigned to welcome at least one patient in the first year, then to increase the numbers as appropriate. A scripted greeting, an outline of the limits of the staff person's authority, and follow-up forms for major problems discovered in rounds are all provided as part of a short training program. Staff members are instructed on things they should not do and where they should turn for help, not unlike the information that volunteers receive. It's a wonderful way to sensitize the staff to the real work of the hospital.

A variety of tasks can be assigned to Associates. They can introduce the hospital's values statement card, help orient Customers to their room, distribute service evaluation forms, run errands, and drop in for a brief chat each day of the patient's stay. Associates respond in a commonsense way to what they discover. If they discover a problem, they are given the responsibility of following up within twenty-four hours to make sure it has been resolved.

Customer Satisfaction Teams. Whose job is Customer satisfaction? Associates are the organization's representatives who supply nearly all the Customer's wants and needs. It is incorrect to think that the Customer should be the primary focus of the manager or supervisor. The manager's primary job is to support the Associates as they serve the Customer! Once these roles are clearly understood, the manager's job becomes a lot simpler. In the New American Hospital, Customer satisfaction is delegated to Associates for implementation. Managers then act to assist Associates in doing their job and strengthening their capacities.

A Customer Satisfaction Team (CST) should be set up in each department large enough to support one. At United Hospital, Clarksburg, West Virginia, CSTs identify and coordinate Customer-related issues. The groups are made up of Associates and are chaired by an Associate. A manager acts as a member of the group in the role of team adviser and selects CST members (CST members often nominate later replacements). Unlike a DIG, which lasts for only thirty days, the CST is meant to be a continuing body in each department, and membership rotates in a staggered fashion. CSTs typically consist of three to five people. Initially, the CST focuses on issues that the members know need fixing; i.e., there are usually more than enough problems that need correcting to get started! In time, the group becomes more refined in assessing Customers' needs through satisfaction measures and interdepartmental feedback.

The focus of the group is defined and limited to issues surrounding Customer service, quality, and productivity. Issues such as corporate policy, human resources practices, and the like are not within its scope of authority. Problems are also limited to those that can be fixed within the unit. However, any CST that sees an interdepartmental problem or an overall policy that needs correcting is asked to report its observations to the appropriate parties.

CSTs are perhaps the most difficult portion of the Customer service strategy to implement, but they are also among the most promising. At one hospital, the CST replaced the Unit Planning Committee and had among its members the Quality Assurance representative and the Staff Nurse Council representative. The CST should become the driving committee of each unit and should use the unit's regular communication meetings to review service issues, discuss solutions, and obtain greater participation and buy-in.

Put Back-Room People On-Line. People who have support functions and don't directly come into contact with Customers can easily lose sight of what the business is all about — serving people. McDonald's Corporation has new hired corporate staff spend several weeks working in the restaurants before reporting to their job as an accountant or lawyer, and at least one day per year thereafter. The Walt Disney Company does the same thing. We suggest having new Associates and managers work some period of time with Customers in patient care areas before beginning work in their regular jobs, and at least one day per year thereafter.

A variation on the back-room-to-the-front-line idea is to have Associates exchange places with their counterparts in another department for a day at a time. This allows Associates in departments with in-house Customers to become better acquainted with their Customer departments. Put them in a place where they can see the impact of what they do. If a Customer has a complaint about food quality, let the person who made the food hear it directly.

Managing Physicians' Accounts

No one needs to be told that physicians are special Customers. The key to establishing strong, positive relationships with them is in responding quickly to improve the place where they practice their profession. Experience shows that once the sources of physicians' complaints have been identified and resolved, they are even more willing to tell you what they would like (as opposed to only telling you what they dislike). Most doctors who complain do so because no system exists to capture their input and solve their problems; the system only reacts to pressure. The goal of this part of the strategy is to *manage* the physician-hospital relationship.

Account management is a simple commonsense way to build the business through strong relationships with the physicians. With strong relationships, physicians will also go out of their way to help refer another doctor or provide support for a project of yours in the future. *I do not advise surveying physicians.* They are already surveyed too much by other organizations and market researchers. A formal survey usually isn't needed to find out what you need to know. Simply ask: "What can we do to make it easier to practice your profession at our place?"

Assign responsibility for physicians' account management to the managers with whom they interact the most. In some cases, assigning the responsibility to nurse managers may be a good idea, since they supervise the staff the doctors interact with. Schedule the initial meeting at the physician's office, and ask for suggestions to improve things. Then get at least one of those problems solved — fast! There probably won't be any difficulty scheduling subsequent meetings, and physicians will call their account managers directly to get problems solved or to place new ideas in the hopper. This idea seems to work equally well for improving the hospital's relationship with the physician's office staff.

Ask the doctor to call his or her account manager directly. The system needs to allow the account manager to place internal calls to different departments that were previously contacted by the doctor. It aggravates doctors to have to make multiple contacts within the hospital. It's not the Customer's job to make the organization respond to their needs — it's our job. Doctors can also be instructed to go to their account managers with problems instead of calling the hospital president. This means that account managers must be empowered to cut across the organization.

Setting Standards and Measuring Results

Excellent organizations establish 95.0 to 99.9 percent Customer satisfaction as a performance standard and take swift corrective action whenever this level is not met. (With this standard, a minimum of 95 percent of Customers would rate the hospital as Good or Excellent on a four-point scale, where two of the adjectives are clearly positive and two are clearly negative.) What are we to make of American hospitals' usual Customer-satisfaction ratings that range between 80 and 85 percent? The number may sound acceptable, but the reality is that these are losing organizations. Hospitals often think they are doing better than they actually are because scaling error distorts the real picture or because not asking the right questions produces skewed results.

The 95 percent minimum standard is based on the finding that 92 percent is necessary just to stay even; because the dissatisfied 8 percent talk to so many others, at 92 percent satisfaction you are merely staying even with them. To win, an organization has to be achieving at some point above 92 percent.

Executives who set standards this high are helping to create a climate of achievement. Knowing that we can meet such a demanding standard becomes a source of pride and motivation, and failure to meet the standard becomes a powerful source of change energy, knocking down resistance to the needed improvements.

Fixing the Rub Points

A patient entering the hospital in pain and discomfort is often required to go through a lengthy admissions process, while all he or she wants is to lie down and be made comfortable. At that moment, the organization is not responding to the Customer's needs. The call light goes on, but is not answered for ten minutes. At that moment, the organization is being judged, rightly or wrongly, as uncaring about its Customer. If the organization "delivers the goods" at that moment, it passes the test of excellence. If it doesn't, a dissatisfied Customer is born.

An important strategy for any successful organization is to identify every interaction where the Customer rubs up against the system (what Jan Carlzon calls "moments of truth") and needs some form of response or accommodation from the organization.[1] What happens in these thousands of individual transactions is critical to the business. Once the interaction points are identified, irritations or disappointments can be smoothed out or removed. This approach also means attempting to meet any needs that are not now being satisfied by changing the system so that Customers benefit in the future.

One solution is to establish and enforce housewide standards of performance (SOPs). Managers need to ask two key questions: What is important to our Customers? When is consistency important to our Customers? The answers may provide a list of areas for the establishment of housewide SOPs:

- *Area appearance.* The hospital should look as good as a Marriott Hotel. Managers should clean up any clutter and dust in their areas.
- *Telephone answering.* All telephones are to be answered courteously within three rings.
- *Customer waiting.* Acknowledge arrival within fifteen seconds and follow up every ten minutes until service is provided.
- *Call lights.* Call lights should be answered within one minute 95 percent or more of the time.
- *Problem response time.* Physician-identified problems are responded to with an action plan within twenty-four hours or one business day.
- *Respect.* The standard is living the Golden Rule. Tactful follow-up is required on all violations. Repeated violations are subject to corrective action.

What other SOPs should be established housewide or within departments? What priority should each SOP have?

Beware the Questionnaire

Effective postservice satisfaction monitoring can be useful, but beware the questionnaire. Avoid the danger of substituting survey results for making changes in the reality seen by your Customers. Surveys are only a means of gathering information — often too late for it to be acted upon. Customers don't care about surveys; they care about the level of service they receive!

Managers' focus should be on resolving service shortcomings, and on taking action to make improvements in existing systems. A walking tour duplicating the Customer's journey through your system often turns up items that need correction. Ask yourself these questions during your tour:

- Is the area clean?
- Is service prompt?
- Is the staff courteous?
- Is the staff happy?
- Do patients and visitors receive orientation information?
- Is the room or service available promptly?
- Is the temperature comfortable?
- Is the food quality good?
- Are the physicians concerned? Are they courteous?
- Did the staff clearly explain the patient's medical care and condition?
- Are postcare instructions clear and helpful?
- Are staff members understanding?
- What is the overall impression?

Unless we work at it, "operational blindness" will occur. This blindness keeps us from seeing our department as it is because it is so familiar to us: our senses don't respond to what we see. *Surveys are no substitute for using common sense and viewing your operations through the Customer's eyes.*

Creating Customer Segment Surveys

Postservice satisfaction measures need to cover four different populations: inpatient, outpatient, emergency department, and outpatient surgery. Each survey should be accompanied by a written statement from the CEO and should be designed so that it contains both open- and closed-ended questions. Computer-scannable forms allow for quicker processing. Open-ended questions may be changed as needed to further investigate specific issues.

Surveys should be given to Customers at either discharge (inpatient and outpatient surgery) or registration (outpatient and emergency). Surveys may be either completed immediately after service and deposited in drop boxes or completed at home and returned by mail in an accompanying postage-paid envelope. Provisions need to be made for critical Customer segments. For example, many emergency room patients are subsequently admitted as inpatients.

Processing of the surveys needs to be centralized to ease collection and reporting. Results are reported on a monthly basis for individual units as well as for the entire hospital. Depending on patient flow, less frequent bimonthly or quarterly reports might be more appropriate. The results should be the first item on the agenda of meetings and the subject of regular management reviews. If severe or common issues are identified for further study, minisurveys or focus groups can be used to obtain more detailed information.

Posting Satisfaction Measures in All Departments

There is no more important feedback than Customer satisfaction. A number of New American Hospitals post a Customer Satisfaction Index (CSI) in each department. Derived from a number of questions relevant to that department's operation, it reduces weekly ratings from Customers to a single data point that is plotted on a graph large enough to be read across the room and that shows the current percentage of patient satisfaction.

Evaluation by In-House Customers

Quantifying the satisfaction levels of the organization's external Customers is important, but what about the departments that serve internal Customers? This important part of the Customer-satisfaction strategy ensures that the people serving external Customers are well supported by their "behind-the-lines" troops.

St. Joseph Hospital, Houston, Texas, uses an in-house customer evaluation that measures in-house Customer satisfaction across the seven KRAs and establishes the 95 percent standard. These surveys are used to generate departmental satisfaction ratings. Visual measures are then posted to spread the word to

Partners (their term for Associates) about the importance of internal Customer satisfaction.

I recommend that these ratings not be immediately tied to the managers' initial merit-and-evaluation review. The idea is to give managers time to straighten problems out themselves. Ratings should not be tied to merit pay until the system has been shaken down. Different tactics can be used to improve relations between in-house customers and suppliers, or to smooth friction between units. One is the "Walk a Mile in My Shoes" program. This allows an Associate or manager to work in another department and see how the interaction between departments looks from the "other side." This can be done on a weekly or monthly basis, with walker honors rotating among department members.

Note

1. J. Carlzon, *Moments of Truth* (New York: Ballinger, 1987).

5

The
Quality-Productivity-Innovation
Equation

None of us is as smart as all of us.
— Ray Kroc
Founder of McDonald's

Getting the work out is essential in a business that operates nonstop around the calendar. And it takes a lot of ideas to get the work done, get it done right, and get it done fast. This chapter will look at the twin challenges of productivity and quality and will examine the *Total Quality Management (TQM)* controversy. The core truth is that quality and productivity come from people, and from how they are allowed to function. The main avenue by which people can bring greater brainpower to bear in small groups will be found in the section called "Do It Groups." With these groups operating, the organization is ready to go into high gear; it stimulates innovation by using an *idea engine*, a supercharged suggestion system. Finally, several cases demonstrate how to finance the creativity the New American Hospital unleashes.

Productivity, Quality, and the TQM Controversy

A lot is being written about productivity and quality management these days. Let's be clear about what productivity is and is not.

Defining Productivity and Quality

Productivity (P) is the ratio expressed by the formula

84

$$P = \text{Output/Input/Time, Quality considered}$$

Output refers to the KRA outputs for which each department is responsible. Key outputs are the only ones that count. We're not interested in producing nonessential work, reports, or meetings. One way to improve productivity is to stop doing trivial work and focus on the right work, the work that counts. Another way is to work harder so that more output is achieved (for the few who are dogging it, this *is* the answer!).

Input refers to manpower, money, minutes, methods, machines, morale, and materials. These are the seven Ms. For ease of use, it's better to primarily focus on manpower — the full-time equivalents (FTEs) or worker-hours required. One way to get more productivity in this part of the formula is to reduce the number of FTEs. That logic works up to a certain point. The real way to accomplish it, however, is to find a way to give people the ability to *do more work in the same amount of time*. This is possible if they are given more training (thus not making mistakes that have to be done over) or better tools. In doing things differently people have figured out a way to work smarter.

Time is the period in which the output amount is compared to the input amount. Because we can compare the output-input ratio for different time periods, it is possible to chart this information to see whether productivity is increasing or decreasing. When more output is achieved per FTE, efficiency has been increased. When there is less output per FTE, efficiency has been decreased. When the same amount of output is done in less time, we have found a way to work faster.

Quality considered stands for the desired level of quality. It's possible to be highly productive but produce junk. Poor quality is not what hospitals want, it's not what Customers want, and it's not what Associates or managers want. Yet there is a real quality problem in hospitals. *Quality* has many meanings, but the two most important ones are doing things in an error-free way and doing them in such a way that Customers are satisfied. Remember that productivity is a subset of quality. *First* we decide what level of quality we want in the work we do and in the kind of organization we work in; *then* we go to work to solve the productivity problems. When we focus on quality, we have decided to work better.

All these definitions are helpful. The summary prescription that comes from them is: *For the work that's worth doing, work harder, smarter, faster, and better.*

Quality and Speed, Not Cost, Are the Keys to Success

American managers in industries overrun by the Japanese found it difficult to accept the idea that quality and speed, not cost, were the keys to success. The correct strategy is to focus first on driving excellence up: then costs will drop. Hospitals are going at it backward. If they focus on intensifying quality, costs will become manageable.

A related concept is that in some cases, being able to move things through the system more quickly is equal to or more important than quality. Time-based competition means that we might not have to do things any differently than we do them now, just faster. Indeed, many Customer complaints are simply requests to reduce wait times.

Additional costs appear as the organization retools to provide higher levels of quality. This is not an argument for quality at any cost, but a recognition that quality improvement requires investment. "You have to spend money to make money," as the old saying goes. What this investment is going to yield is an improvement in the practices and steps needed to drive quality up. It is also important for the organization to realize that cost containment must never come at the expense of quality. Quality is the investment that creates the greatest opportunity to drive costs down.

Continuous Improvement Is the Only Kind

Initially, the biggest obstacle to getting a problem solved is that people may not see it as a problem, asking "If it's not broke, why fix it?" There are two answers: "Everything is broke!" and its corollary, "If it's not broke, fix it anyway!" Every form, practice, system, and procedure is imperfect. Because of the rapid pace of change, we cannot be successful by doing next year what we did last year. In a rapidly changing and imperfect world, everything we are doing needs to be fixed, revised, improved—even scrapped. There is no need to be defensive about the way we do things now because we're about to improve everything! Remember, everything is in need of improvement.

Once the old hospital was willing to admit that something did need fixing, it got caught up in the perfection trap. It didn't see that just as nothing is perfect now, there can also be no perfect solutions. There can never be more than partial solutions, partial answers, and partial improvements. Today's "perfect answer" is just the best we can do at the time. What does this mean? It means that managers should be content with partial answers and add improvements into the system as soon as possible. Do the best you can today, make those changes now, and come back to a project for improvements later. Thus there is a bias for action, not the bias for inaction for which most hospitals are committee-famous. The rule here is that everything is in need of improvement, *continuously*.

In the New American Hospital, Associates and managers study a problem, make their best decision, implement it quickly, and don't wait for a perfection that never comes. As a consequence, a lot more change happens. The New American Hospital establishes an organizational culture that pushes to keep improving. It views change as a continuous flow rather than a discrete event. The great secret of excellence is improvement today, not "perfection" tomorrow.

However, continuous improvement does not necessarily mean never-ending or unceasing improvement. It is possible to improve things past the point of their having value to the Customer. As one wise hospital leader said, "We're interested in improving continuously and adding value that the market is willing to pay for." A number of American manufacturers, finding that improving past the point of Customer acceptance is fruitless, have been reducing efforts to ceaselessly vary or improve their offerings. We don't need forty more varieties of corn chips, or another hundred car models. In all these things,

staying close to the Customer is the best defense against
overimprovement.

What Productivity and Quality Are Not

Quality and productivity are not pushing people around. Telling people to work harder or better isn't effective. They're not
working at low levels because they choose to. Most people want
to work both hard and well. Studies of productivity and quality
show that only about 20 percent of the failure to produce quality
and productivity is within the workers' direct control. Eighty
percent lies outside of the workers' control, tied up in poor
systems, policies, practices, and "the way things are done."

Quality and productivity are not the ability to meet
JCAHO standards. In recent years the hospital industry has
added quality assurance departments, failing to understand
how management really takes place. The concept that quality
can effectively be monitored, measured, controlled, or directed
from a staff department after the care has been given was another will-of-the-wisp JCAHO requirement.

Quality can't be controlled by inspections from an outside agency. The thoughtful person understands that quality is
everybody's job. The New American Hospital puts control over
quality into the hands of each worker, educates them in quality-
improvement methods, and creates measurement systems so
that all performers understand how their work measures up.
The idea that quality can be achieved by having an outsider
come around every three years is a myth and a travesty of logic.

Quality and productivity are not simply TQM programs.
Quality and its related issues of Customer service, cost, productivity, and human utilization are infinitely greater than a TQM
program. And quality can't be achieved solely by a TQM effort.
The rush to install these programs in old hospitals will meet
with failure in many cases, a failure caused by amateurs who are
unwilling to manage their organization correctly and do the
hard work of total management.

Total Management, Not Total Quality Management

As hospitals attempt to alter their approach to management, they repeatedly fall into the trap of partial strategies and piecemeal change. Total Quality Management (TQM) is the latest remedial fad, the latest entrant in the long parade of programs in guest relations, cost containment, quality circles, stress management, and nurse recruitment that have been tried and failed. Unfortunately, the prognosis for TQM is no better; it is yet another "program of the month" to afflict hospital managers.

TQM and other related approaches, such as Continuous Quality Improvement and Quality Improvement programs, represent both a philosophy and a methodology for solving work system problems. While various schools of thought and differences of application are represented by such older names as W. Edwards Deming, Joseph Juran, and Philip Crosby and new-wave thinkers like Masaaki Amai, they all recommend the use of small groups of people who are close to the problem and equipped with such management-engineering and problem-solving tools as fishbone charts, Gantt charts, variance analysis, flowcharts, traffic diagrams, histograms, and basic statistics. Their primary emphasis is on the quality issues surrounding an organization's products and services, along with the related issues of Customer satisfaction and feedback. While the value of cultural change and a positive support climate are acknowledged by TQM proponents, these elements are presumed to be largely present, a false assumption in the case of the old hospital model.

Why TQM Programs Risk Failure

I do not make my dire predictions for TQM and other quality efforts because I am against these programs. I am fully behind the efforts of those who seek to improve quality in the kind of systematic and organized ways that TQM represents. The problem arises when TQM encounters the quietly hostile atmosphere of the old hospital's corporate culture. This nonsupportive climate makes it almost impossible for the innovative wave that TQM can represent to exist. Think of TQM primarily as a set of tools and problem-solving methods. The old hospital says, "I'll buy the tools, but I don't think I'll let the workmen rebuild the house!"

Is TQM a wrong approach? No. What's wrong is that many hospitals do not display the conditions of change readiness that will allow it to succeed. Hospitals need the tools and approaches that TQM offers, but old hospitals represent a counterculture to the positive assumptions about people made by the quality move- ment, and the old hospital's approaches to management will not provide the proper foundation in which TQM can flourish. Hence my conclusion that this initiative will largely fail.

At the time of this writing, symptoms of program rejec- tion are already being seen in hospitals. They indicate a corpo- rate culture that is nonsupportive of the help TQM could offer:

- Implementation that is too slow and extended time frames
- Little in the way of early business results
- Too much orientation to data, studies, and go-slow signals
- Lack of buy-in from an already overburdened staff
- A consultant-dependent attitude that means the program is not easily self-sustainable
- An orientation toward process instead of outcomes

Given the substantial cost of a TQM effort, it's essential for hospitals to capitalize on their investment. TQM programs take twice as long to implement, require more managerial hand holding, and experience uneven implementation in organiza- tions that have not undergone previous cultural renewal. How- ever, when Total Management approaches were done first, TQM became a natural outgrowth, the next phase of the organiza- tion's pursuit of excellence. Thus, simply by reversing the se- quence of organizational change, it becomes possible for quality-improvement efforts to succeed. But what is Total Management?

The Need for Total Management

The quality target is best hit by installing a New American Hospital model first, one that creates the kind of supportive environment in which TQM can flourish. TQM programs have worked very successfully in the new hospital, in part because of the change readiness that such an organization fosters. Without this framework, TQM is too narrow a technique, and it cannot stand alone. Whether it is in vogue or not, changing the organization's culture and developing a strong management team is the prerequisite to reaching the heart of quality, Customer, and productivity issues.

It would be nice to be able to focus on quality efforts alone, but the hospital is not a program; it is a continuously functioning mechanism that has to be managed in its totality. Only when the hospital is managed correctly by seeing the wholeness of achieving all seven KRAs can quality concerns be adequately addressed. Can quality ever happen if *people growth* does not? Can it flourish if *Customer service* does not? Will TQM work in an organization if issues of *economics* and *productivity* are not addressed? How can an organization with little in the way of *innovation* or flow of ideas be successful in improving its quality? And if the *organizational climate* is sour, will people show the gusto that quality requires? Clearly, all KRAs must be dealt with, for their dynamic interaction is the only way possible to improve organizational performance.

Which Approach Produces Better Results?

More than a philosophical argument, the basic question in management always remains the same: Where are the results? Experience in the New American Hospital shows both faster and greater results in terms of addressing quality and Customer issues. While most TQM programs counsel patience and expect results to be years in coming, Lima Memorial Hospital in Lima, Ohio, was able to conduct four hundred DIGs in the first sixteen months of its change effort and achieve a net savings of $2 million.[1] It's important to recognize that TQM approaches represent a significant step up the ladder but that they aren't the best first step. It is possible to achieve higher and faster quality results when TM approaches provide a foundation for TQM efforts.

Targeting Priorities for Improvement

What are the highest priorities for improvement? While everything needs to be improved, some items are more essential than
others. The best way to determine which items to choose is to ask
Associates, Customers, and managers what they'd like improved
and start with their high priorities.

     In addition to the list generated in-house, here are some
areas you may want to consider in targeting improvements. They
yield tremendous results because of the influence they have on
other factors (e.g., a meeting management system), or because of
the large effect even a small project can have (five seconds saved
in making a salad times ten thousand salads per year).

     Improve Patient Care Systems. One commonsense way to
attack productivity and quality issues is to start with what the
patient needs and work out from there. Not only is that correct
from the perspective of business and values, but it also taps into
the motivational needs of Associates who find their greatest
satisfaction in helping others. "Do it for the patients," is like a war
cry. So let's start with the target's bull's-eye.

- *Solve the problem of delays.* Customers hate delays in admis-
  sion, lying on gurneys in the hall, and being moved from
  room to room. There are answers to those problems. Attacking wait times usually reveals a host of underlying projects to
  work on. And remember, we'll take even half an answer!
- *Use paraprofessionals wherever possible.* Never use a registered
  nurse to do a job an aide can do. If the aides could do it, but
  don't know how, then train them!
- *Invest in transport robotics and new biotechnology.* If nurses are
  running errands to and from the lab, X-Ray, and Central
  Supply, your hospital is failing to use twenty-five-year-old
  transport technology. Robot boxes follow magnetic tape,
  sense obstacles, and get the job done. And find out if the lab
  is fully automated.
- *Standardize the process of care.* Start by standardizing nursing
  procedures that vary by shift, unit, or individual nurse.
  Standardize where the supplies are kept on each unit so that

staff always know where to find them. Start standardizing some of the technology to get better mass purchasing prices and fewer replacement pieces to stock in inventory. Get Pharmacy started on reducing the too-wide range of pharmacological products. Allow Purchasing to lower the number of items in inventory by helping the hospital to standardize tools and materials.

Invest in Tools. A reliable rule of thumb is to buy any and all tools that represent a savings in employee time. This rule holds true about 90 percent of the time. When you compare the cost of a tool to the cost of the time an Associate needs to do the work without the tool, over the expected lifetime of that tool, it's cost-effective to buy the tool.

Could your people be more productive if they had more tools? I have heard horror stories of nurses with too few blood pressure cuffs and stethoscopes. The organizations save a nickel and then spend hundreds of dollars in lost labor time while nurses hunt for cuffs. Meanwhile the patient is having cardiac arrest! The Japanese automated their automobile plants years before American automakers. Are they better workers, or do they just have better tools?

Ask managers and Associates what tools they need. The wish list would stagger Santa! Get started on making it come true. While you're at it, don't buy cheap tools. Forget what Purchasing says and listen to what the worker wants. There's a convincing case for the idea that the initial savings of cheaper tools mask shorter lifetimes and greater maintenance costs.

Computerize! No more powerful tool has come along in recent years than the computer. This technology is not going to go away, yet its penetration into the American hospital is low. When it comes to improving productivity and quality, this is one of the big guns. Studies show that most executives don't know how to use computers and therefore don't understand what their value can be. And I'm not even talking about mainframes, but the workstations and personal computers that put the tool into the hands of the people.

Include Performance Planning. The objective of performance planning, a simple form of management by objectives, is to clearly delineate each job position and to set in motion a quarterly work plan that will specify what is to be accomplished in that period. As Peter Drucker wrote, "One either manages by objectives, or one does not manage." Studies clearly show that organizations without quarterly performance plans, such as hospitals, do not produce nearly as much as those with them. New American Hospitals report that their productivity is greatly enhanced when work teams focus on the right kind of outputs. Exhibit 5.1 shows a sample form that is used to lay out the work.

The forms are filled out by managers and some professional/technical Associates and reviewed by the management. Differences of opinion are then negotiated in a joint meeting. The amount of preparation time required will vary by job but a form usually requires an hour for an Associate to complete. The review time with the manager typically averages thirty minutes per Associate, a modest amount of time for creating a management tool that will control work for the next ninety days.

Position focus is designed to clearly identify the major objectives or results that a particular job is to accomplish. Many job descriptions become lengthy recitals of various tasks and duties rather than a specification of what the job is actually supposed to accomplish. A usual problem is that fewer than half of manager-Associate pairs can agree on 50 percent of the job elements! In Figure 5.1 an Associate describes his job as having certain elements, but the manager thinks that he should be doing a different cluster of events. Where these two boxes overlap, there is agreement and congruence. In these areas. the Associate is doing what the manager thinks he should be doing.

The Associate also thinks he should be doing other tasks; this causes the manager to wonder why the Associate is choosing those tasks over the ones the manager thinks are important. Left unmanaged, the expectations that each has of the job lead to blind alleys, unnecessary work, frustration and conflict. The first function of planned performance is to reach agreement about exactly what the job is and how much time and effort the job incumbent should be spending on doing it.

Exhibit 5.1. Performance Plan.

Planned Performance

MANSYS℠ The Integrated Management System

Associate _____ Title _____

Manager _____ Date _____

A. Position Focus		B. Work Plan						
Key Functions/Responsibilities (What's the job?)	Weight (What %)	Projects/Objectives (What's to be done?)	Priority (A,B,C)	Authority (A,B,C)	Scheduling Start	Scheduling Review	Scheduling Complete	Results/Standards of Performance (How will results be judged?)

Source: C. Sherman, *MANSYS, The Integrated Management System* (Inverness, Ill.: Management House, 1989). Reprinted with permission.

Figure 5.1. Differences in Job Perceptions.

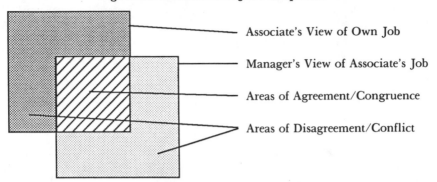

— Associate's View of Own Job

— Manager's View of Associate's Job

— Areas of Agreement/Congruence

— Areas of Disagreement/Conflict

The *work plan* portion of the planned performance program is designed to list the specific projects or tasks that will be undertaken in the current quarter. While the form can be completed on an as-needed basis, experience suggests that sitting down with some discipline every ninety days and mapping out a specific work plan makes the most sense. Lee Iacocca revealed that part of his successful turnaround of Chrysler Corporation came from his belief that he should establish quarterly work objectives for all members of his team. He reasoned that if the shareholders, the investors who own the business, insisted on a quarterly report of earnings to see how the company was doing, that same process of taking a quarterly look at how work was progressing was good enough for him as well.[2]

Productive People—Quality People

Productivity and quality come only from productive and quality people. The prime directive is to free them to do what they already know how to do, and to find ways to help them do more. The most exciting illustration of this is the story of how hospital workers are succeeding in small groups.

Having Associates Control Their Own Work

As organizational renewal unfolds, Associates will want to have some control over what is going on in their department. In one hospital, a housekeeping supervisor had previously inspected the areas cleaned by her staff. She changed from this approach by having Associates draw up a list of what should be done in a patient's room. The list was then used as a checklist, which the Associates reviewed for each room they completed. In this way, control was moved from the supervisor to the Associates. When they began to think through what they needed to accomplish, they took more responsibility. Many went back to their completed rooms later in the shift to touch them up so that their work still looked good at the end of the shift; this was above and beyond what their supervisor used to require.

Having Associates Redesign Jobs and Work Systems

Measurement brings problems out in the open. As measurement of productivity, quality, and Customer satisfaction is established, Associates will have suggestions about areas that need to be changed and improved. When problems come to light, individual workers or groups should be assigned the responsibility and given the freedom to redesign work systems. We're not interested in measuring for its own sake; we're interested in measuring so that we can change and improve. The worst possible thing management can do is to give workers feedback, but then say, "Well, you can't change that policy," or "That procedure really isn't in our authority to manage." If you pick up one end of the stick, you also have to pick up the other end.

Increasing Group Efficiency by Regrouping Tasks

Typically, in low-productivity areas, job descriptions are relatively inefficient. Not only are the jobs often stripped of meaning but the work flow doesn't make sense either. Instead of rewriting job descriptions, one manager identified all the necessary tasks and activities that had to be accomplished in the department and then made a decision as to who would be primarily and secondarily responsible for the execution of those tasks. The matrix she designed became a *unit* job description. She recognized that targeting responsibility was a secondary concern; it

was the unit job description, the unit work list, that really had to
be managed. Who did each task within the unit was of less
importance. Under this concept, it's possible to rethink the
whole question of who should be doing a task, because it is clear
at a glance how everyone interacts in order to get the work of the
department accomplished.

Cross-Training Between Shifts and Units

An evaluation of how well a hospital is achieving prime targets
will immediately expose problems between shifts or departments. One of the best ways to get at these problems is by cross-
training. This is not: "Let's visit them for a day to understand
their operations." It's a more intensive concept: "Let's train in
their area so that we can understand how they do their work and
see how their system fits in with our work flow." When an understanding develops between the two departments or shifts, it
then becomes productive to set up a task force to deal with the
problem. Contrast that approach to what we sometimes see:
the establishment of a task force when no one understands what
the other area does. The task force is unprepared and not ready
to do its work.

Changing Performance with Measured Feedback

Measurement and feedback change behavior. Organizations
and individuals often continue to do inappropriate things because they don't know how they're doing. One way to change
behavior is to set a standard, show people how to achieve it, and
establish a feedback system that shows them when the standard
isn't being met. Both individual pride and a sensible reward
system will provide the motivation to change what people are
doing.

   Communication Centers—Getting It Out in the Open. The
Communication Center (see Exhibit 5.2) is a bulletin board
located in each department that serves to keep visible the work
flow and other items people need to be familiar with in order to
do their jobs well. The cardinal rule is that people should be

Exhibit 5.2. Communication Center.

What We Stand for	The Plan of Attack	Customer Expectations and Needs	Results
Values statement	Quarterly work plan	Service expectations and needs	Criticisms or kudos
Where We're Going	Amendments		Customer ratings
Strategic objectives	Changed priorities	Focus group notes	Productivity statistics
		Key standards of performance	Budget information
Views	*News*	*Suggestions and Ideas*	*General*
Policy announcements	Major business news		
Changes in procedure	New developments		
Supervisory directives			

Source: C. Sherman, *MANSYS, The Integrated Management System* (Inverness, Ill.: Management House, 1989). Reprinted with permission.

allowed to know anything they want to know, as long as it does not violate any other person's interests. Nothing is to be hidden, including budgets, the organization's strategic plan, and complaints about the department. An *open* work society is necessary for an *improved* work society.

What do your people want to know? What should they know? The manager who openly displays information is not going to have to worry about being thought of as secretive. Ask yourself: Would you be better off if you could identify this kind of information with your boss? Core items might include:

1. *Direction giving*
   - A copy of the organization's values statement
   - The major objectives for the year as stated in the strategic plan
   - A copy of the current quarter's planned performance work objectives

2. *Measures of results*
    - A list of the department's standards of performance for Customer interaction
    - Monthly and year-to-date measures of Customer satisfaction, productivity, and budget outcomes
    - All kudos and criticisms received
3. *Current events and changes*
    - The current issue of the supervisory newsletter
    - All general notices
4. *Associates' inputs*
    - A place to list questions, comments, and suggestions (an alternative way to do this would be to set up a departmental suggestion box)
5. *Optional items*
    - The Associates' newsletter
    - A segment to post items for sale and other matters of general interest

Post all comments, including complaints that Customers submit. Putting these "good news, bad news" pictures onto the Communication Center board gives us a reading on our performance and the Customer's perception of our performance. There is a tendency in poorly performing organizations to hide the dirty laundry and not to openly discuss a Customer's complaint. This becomes covered over with such labels as "confidentiality" and "protecting other people's feelings." We can't stop the problem until we deal openly with the issues. If the Customer is unhappy we'd better fix it, and the sooner the issue is on the table the better.

Posting Productivity, Quality, and Customer Measures. Always post a Customer Satisfaction Index (CSI). The CSI is derived from a number of questions and then converted to a 100-point scale. When one head nurse posted this number the first week, it was 82 points. She didn't explain it. She didn't find fault. She didn't hold a meeting. She simply created a large graph. The next week she posted the next number. By the third week, there was open questioning and discussion about what the numbers meant. No group of people with any pride would be satisfied with an 82 rating out of 100 points. Building on their dissatisfaction with the score, the head nurse led them to solve the problems that had created the low rating—feedback had changed unit behavior.

Other measures of productivity and quality should also be posted. Measurement is the great tool that leads to higher productivity and quality, if the support climate of the New American Hospital is present. Some general rules of thumb regarding measures are:

- Establish two to four measures per unit, because each one provides only a partial picture.
- Identify baselines so that seasonal trends don't throw you.
- Display the measures in graph form on the Communication Center board.

The New American Hospital isn't very interested in comparisons to other hospitals or to national and regional statistics. The true measures compare the present to the organization's past achievements. Are we beating our numbers?

Do It Groups

While all writers and practitioners advocate the value of small groups as the primary vehicle for participative decision making, a number of divergent views are now emerging about how these groups should function. Others have written extensively and well on small-group dynamics and the procedures by which these groups function. My own small contribution is to challenge the view of how fast these groups can successfully operate (a lot faster), and of the total volume of change they can accomplish (a lot more). *Do It Groups* (DIGs) is our name for project teams that meet to solve problems. DIGs are not committees that go on forever and accomplish little or nothing. They are not academic study groups. They are just commissioned to get things done.

DIGs focus on solving a single, specific problem *within thirty days.* The goal is improvement, not perfection, with an emphasis on fast results. Quick implementation of these results can be followed up with successive improvements. To make sure a DIG is not wasting time on unimportant things, it concentrates on problems that are tied to the hospital's mission as expressed in its corporate values and the KRAs.

Multiplying DIGs

This approach has worked extremely well in organizational renewal. In the typical New American Hospital, we begin with about ten groups made up from the sixty department heads. Those groups finish in thirty days, and within two weeks they are reformed and doubled to about twenty DIGs. In the next cycle, there are forty DIGs, with each group having only about 25 percent management representation. The reason for increasing DIGs in this fashion is to have some members who have had at least a little experience, as well as bringing in Associates. The rapid expansion has a twofold purpose: (1) to cascade the change process down into the organization and maximize Associate participation as early as possible and (2) to produce the maximum change as quickly as possible. Producing results is the best way to overcome resistance to change.

At about the second or third cycle, the process begins to multiply almost out of control. In the first twelve months hospitals will complete a number of DIGs equivalent to 50 percent of the total number of Associates they employ. A 2,200-Associate work force in Texas completed 1,050 DIGs; a work force of 900 completed 400!

How a DIG Works

In the early rounds, Associates and managers tend to go after "targets of opportunity," things they see in their line of sight that need fixing. Later on, management is allowed to suggest problem areas where they'd like help, but they do not control the topics. Because Associates want to succeed, they will take general guidance, with wise management getting out of the way!

A DIG sometimes completes its work in one meeting with

a group of people who find a solution to a problem. It does not need to be a formalized group with regular meetings. Or it may take multiple meetings to hammer something out. Ideas for DIGs are suggested to department managers, or alternately to a housewide DIG Coordinator, by individual Associates, management, or even Customers or visitors. Small groups in departments or during seminars often come up with ideas, or ideas might come from news of other excellent organizations. We want all the good ideas we can get.

DIG suggestions are submitted on a DIG Creation Form and reviewed within fourteen days to determine appropriate action. Actions usually take one of the following forms:

- Forward suggestions to key department heads for comment within five days.
- Make individual "just do it" assignments to an Associate if the suggestion does not require a DIG or is clearly within someone's job responsibility.
- Determine that an interdepartmental DIG is needed, clarify the DIG focus, identify the key departments to be involved, and post the DIG for sign-up.
- Determine that a department DIG is needed and assign follow-up to the appropriate management team member. Most DIGs occur within the department.
- Reject the idea due to a lack of feasibility or practicality. Following the command to "never kill an idea," managers are expected to find a way to make a minimum of 90 percent of DIG-processed ideas work. In a number of hospitals, any DIG recommendations that are turned down are reviewed by the CEO. This really keeps the heat on to change the system!

As the DIG begins its work, it is important to zero in on areas where you can make a difference and to avoid letting the focus become too general or global. The DIG Coordinator (or other support person) helps assure that DIG topics are manageable. When a topic appears to be too global, the problem should be broken down into pieces so that several DIGs can address the key components of the larger problem. This feature is a key variation from the idea that one group oversees the process from start to finish. In computerese, we believe that a "coprocessor" route is preferable, and speedier.

Tips for Constructing a DIG

The following are helpful tips to keep in mind when constructing a DIG:[3]

- Never set up a DIG if the task is small enough to be handled by one responsible person.
- Have the DIG chair select two to six other managers or Associates to serve on the DIG. Where possible, it is recommended that there be no more than two managers on a DIG in order to encourage wider participation. Get as many affected parties together as possible, and touch base with others for input as needed.
- Pick a small, doable project, not a complete remake of the organization.
- Set a deadline to find some form of solution within thirty days. Treat the thirty days as the outside limit. On rare occasions the DIG may decide to extend the project for another thirty days.
- If a project is big and complex, set up several DIGs to crunch through it. One DIG is often the source of other future DIGs.
- When the DIG has completed its task, disband the group. Members are then free to participate in other DIGs. Some organizations set a requirement of managerial participation on at least six DIGs a year and Associate participation of one DIG a year, to assure that the organization is continually being prodded.
- Make sure that all members are participating fully. Remove those who are not contributing, calling it a rotation. Recruitment and membership questions should primarily be decided by the DIG itself. Don't let conflicts about the group hold up progress.
- Follow good meeting management practices to make your meetings productive (start on time, follow the agenda, don't let discussions bog down, end on time, etc.).

- Remember that you are after improvement, not perfection. Your mission is not 100 percent of all the things that could be done in some ideal universe, but rather the 60 to 80 percent that are doable now. Make it better and let another group improve it later as needed. Action is the name of the game.

I have had good success with training DIG members in basic DIG procedures, brainstorming skills, and the DO-IT problem-solving sequence explained in the next section. Our goal has been to get people into a successful group experience quickly, increase their confidence, and make them believe in the system by allowing them a piece of the action within the first year. Toward the end of that year, we have DIG members go through a second wave of training in classic TQM tools such as Pareto analysis and decision matrices. This has resulted in much higher learner readiness; the DIG members have come up the learning curve and are ready for more tools. Thus the need for greater sophistication follows the first need for rapid cultural change.

The Problem-Solving Sequence

My spin on the problem-solving sequence designed by others is a play on the action phrase DO-IT:[4]

> Define Problem
> Organize Options
> Implement Solutions
> Track Results

Each step has a defined problem-solving logic, with subsets of questions, and utilizes continuous-improvement tools as appropriate.

Nothing in the use of DIGs precludes using other groups such as task forces, project teams, or committees, but DIGs have proved to be more useful than any other small-group process as a change engine. They create a tidal wave of change, producing both results and esprit de corps.

Revving Up Innovation

We need an idea engine. Medical knowledge is doubling every five years, and it seems as if problems in the health care industry are doubling even faster! The New American Hospital knows that the only answers you're likely to get these days are the ones you create yourself. Where do our in-house ideas come from now? Unfortunately, most come from management. It's not that these folks don't have good ideas and good brains, but they don't have enough of them.

Try this exercise. Fill in the following chart:

	Managers	Associates	Customers
Number of People			
Number of Brains			
Number of Ideas Submitted			
Percentage of Ideas Implemented			

If you can't complete the numbers for Associates and Customers, you're working in an old hospital. In a discussion of why staff isn't listened to, one supervisor said, "My management thinks our people are halfwits." Even if that cynicism were true, with management only 10 percent of the work force, Associates' brainpower would still outdistance management's 5 to 1! As for Customers, if the organization had a way to collect their ideas and involve them in groups, they could transform the organization! We've got the brainpower; we just need a system to utilize it.

In the past, hospitals would sometimes solicit and receive suggestions, then not know what to do with them. They didn't have any way to process the new ideas. In the New American Hospital, the idea engine is a natural outgrowth of the DIG process that is put in place first. Think of the DIG system as a collection of data processors. Once it's built, it's ready to grind through all the ideas that can be generated.

System Benefits

One of the advantages of having all ideas flowing through a central suggestion system is to identify idea clusters that surround certain issues or problems. If six people turn in ideas that are highly similar or related, form them into a DIG.

In one New American Hospital ideas are tracked by topic, quantity, and timing. By seeing what topics are suggested, management can sense where it has the most problems. By counting the number of suggestions, it can judge whether there is enough production of innovation, a manageable output.

The system captures "throw-away ideation." How many times in a meeting have you heard someone say, "What we need is . . ." or "Wouldn't it be great if we . . . ?" These ideas that get lost in the shuffle are assets that are sometimes more valuable than money. With a tracking system, all ideas are entered under the appropriate KRA and descriptor codes for later retrieval.

Driving Change with a Minimum Implementation Rate

Reports from the idea engine track a number of key statistics to judge the health of the system and the value of the ideas that are implemented. A first-year requirement is that managers implement a minimum of 50 percent of the ideas received from Associates. This has proved to be easily achievable, with at least a portion of the initial idea being implemented about 75 percent of the time. This requirement prevents people from saying, "It can't be done." Instead, the cultural pressure is toward "Great idea! Let's do it!" The greatest reward, as judged by Associates, is in seeing their idea implemented.

Input Channels for Suggestions

1. *Revitalize the suggestion box.* The old hospital usually has an employee suggestion box — empty and a butt of jokes. Every-

body knows that suggestion boxes don't work, yet even this old system can be revitalized. In one hospital, supervisors put suggestion boxes in their units. They said to their Associates, "Let's put a box here for anything you want to say. I'll read each comment or suggestion in front of all of you and open up a group discussion. If the idea has some consensus, I'll either make the change on the spot or allow you to discuss further how you might like to handle it." This new approach to an old way of gathering ideas was very successful. It isn't what you do; it's how you do it.

2. *Phone it in.* Set up a telephone extension of an Idea Center that can be reached by dialing IDEA on the telephone. The Idea Center is a secretary who takes down suggestions. Anything that communicates the importance of ideas and speeds their delivery is to be desired. What other channels of idea input can you think of?

3. *Form Customer Councils.* Sometimes called Committees of Excellence, these are focus groups of Customers who have experienced a department's services. A committee is established for each department, meeting on a regular basis to make suggestions for improvement.

4. *Ask visitors.* In one New American Hospital, idea engine forms were placed in each waiting room. The form said that the organization was engaged in an improvement process and was looking for good ideas to improve its system. Directions were given for depositing the form and routing it back for action. Contact information was requested in case of additional questions. This information was also useful in identifying people who were particularly articulate and possibly good candidates for the Committees of Excellence or for serving on a DIG.

5. *Surveys of physicians.* What happens to all the ideas that come from physicians' complaints now? Do we really need to run yet another survey, only to have the hospital, once again, do nothing with the information? Respond and be aggressive toward these problems.

Reward All Suggestion Steps

Since behavior follows rewards, send a thank-you note for each idea received and add a lapel pin in the shape of a light bulb. Employees who send in ten ideas can receive a campaign button, "Member of the Brain Trust." Or give an Associate a shovel pin for serving on a DIG, a gold shovel for serving on ten DIGs, and a board or presidential salute for twenty-five! For each idea implemented, give one hundred bonus points toward awards out of a merchandise catalog. You get the idea. Devise a system based on the behaviors that are needed and that are within your budget.

Finding Resources for Creativity

"We can't afford to do it" is the oldest ploy used to resist making change. To break this barrier, assign the vice president of finance to create discretionary funds for off-budget projects that need initial developmental capital to make them doable. Later, they can be added to the normal cost picture. To assist this thinking, track the estimated first-year value of each DIG; this shows the average return on investment. The universal finding of New American Hospitals is that returns exceed costs and do so within the first year.

One example is that of the Appalachia Cluster of the Sunbelt Health System (Seventh Day Adventist). This is a group of four small rural hospitals that undertook a joint effort to go through renewal. They have a total of 1,300 Associates, and in the first eight months they completed 679 DIGs and had 127 more in process. Figure 5.2 shows their results for the first twelve months. Measurements were done by each organization; they report that the cost picture was quite complete, but that only tangible returns were used, gains where hard dollars could be measured. Costs included management development, consultant costs, time costs of DIG meetings, implementation costs of DIG recommendations, and all other costs traceable to the renewal effort. Intangible gains, such as morale improvement or

Figure 5.2. Appalachia Cluster Return on Investment, 9/1/91–9/1/92.

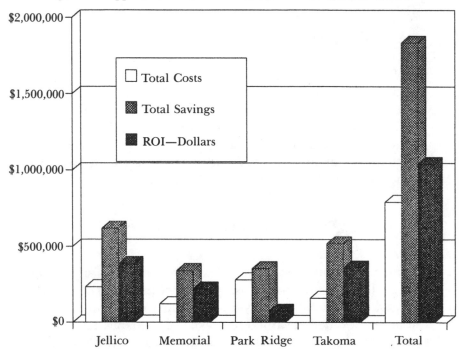

Customer satisfaction, were also obtained, but are not shown in the figure.

Two aspects of this picture are noteworthy. First, the change-model sequence of making managerial and cultural change first, rapidly followed by the formation of DIG groups, was successful in demonstrating that organizational renewal represents a good financial risk. Second, the model was sufficiently stable and predictable for all four organizations to achieve success with it, though the rate of return varied.

A second illustration further helps to answer the concern about whether organizational change is financially helpful. Figure 5.3 shows tangible returns of $195,000 for Northern Illinois

Medical Center (NIMC) in the first year of their reengineering effort. This was a private study commissioned by the hospital from the University of Wisconsin Hospitals and Clinics.[5] Although 164 DIGs were done in the start-up year, only 76 could pass the criteria used by the researchers to show tangible, measurable gains. Again, the model shows an actual positive first-year picture, followed by projections of costs and returns in the subsequent four-year period. Like TQM advocates, I believe that returns are increasingly better with time because the organization becomes more and more efficient. However, unlike TQM proponents, I believe that unless returns can be produced early, there is a risk that the change initiative may be showing early signs of ineffectiveness. TQM says be patient, the results will come in time. But tough-minded executives prefer TM, which gets results both now and in the future.

The Wisconsin researchers then tried to rate the value of the intangibles produced by the other 88 DIGs which concluded during the first year. Using a scale of their own devising, and making an effort to control for positive group bias, they found the results pictured in Figure 5.4, where almost 80 percent of the hard-to-measure DIGs had produced some substantial savings of improvement. In spite of the measurement problem, it is important to keep in mind that intangible results are real and substantial.

As powerful as the outcomes of the small groups were at NIMC, it is important to note that these results were obtained because of the change climate created by Paul Laudick, the hospital's president. More than 95 percent of the 1,126 ideas submitted by Associates, Customers, and management in the first two years of the change process were implemented! Laudick created the expectation — the positive demand — that the organization respond to the innovation that was waiting to be born.

Besides using DIG processors to generate gains through innovation, the other major approach to freeing up scarce capital is to cut costs. The New American Hospital knows that cutting costs by simply slashing budgets is a recipe for disaster. Cost containment is a legitimate need and a requirement of good productivity management, but it has to be accomplished

Figure 5.3. Northern Illinois Medical Center: Return on Investment from Seventy-Six DIGs.

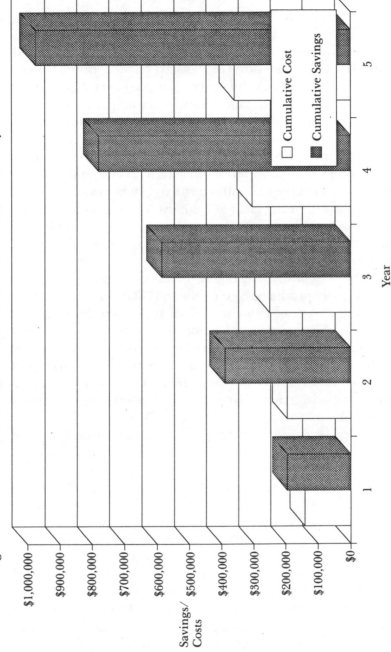

Note: Return on Investment of DIGs done in year 1 showing actual first-year return and projected value in following years.

Figure 5.4. Northern Illinois Medical Center: Ratings of DIG Impact and Quality.

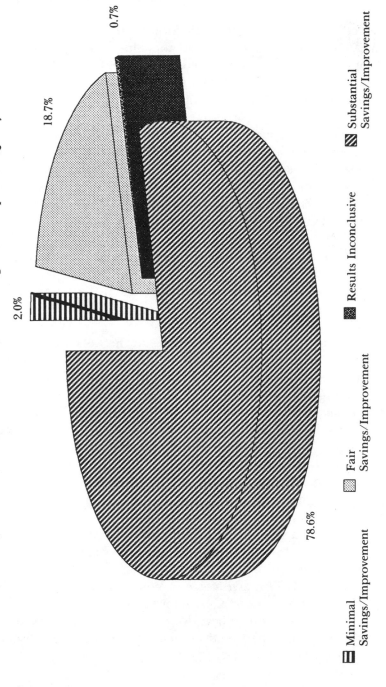

0.7%

18.7%

2.0%

78.6%

⊞ Minimal
Savings/Improvement

▒ Fair
Savings/Improvement

▓ Results Inconclusive

▨ Substantial
Savings/Improvement

in a creative way. We must tell the organization to contain costs, reduce operating expenses, and look for new ways of doing things. One effective way to reduce costs is to attack waste. A cost-containment exercise can be given to each department, with questions like the following:[6]

- *Organizational management.* If you were in the shoes of your president, what are three opportunities for cost improvement you would insist upon before a new annual budget was approved?
- *Departmental management.* Is departmental deadwood being attended to? Are there too many "blockers and complainers" here?
- *Information, forms, and supplies.* The generation of reports is costly. Identify reports that can be either shortened and made more concise or amputated from the management system.
- *Systems and procedures.* Find unnecessary delays. Where is cost generated because of bottlenecks in the work flow, inaccurate procurement lead time, poor scheduling, and so on? Where can you minimize delays, frequently recurring "emergencies," missing information, and so on?
- *Human utilization and development.* Employee turnover is costly. In your organization, where has employee turnover been a costly problem? What changes are needed to decrease this expensive turnover?
- *Technology and tools.* Where are tools, big or little, needed in order to do things more cheaply, quicker, or better?
- *Time management.* Where are you generating unnecessary costs through duplication of efforts, duplication of time being spent, or overlapping assignments between people or functions?
- *Investment by KRA to reduce costs.* Where can you reduce costs by spending more on Customer service?
- *Planning and control.* Where do you waste effort and resources by having unclear direction, lack of planning, or an absence of priorities?

Provide an incentive by promising that the department will get some percentage of the amount saved. In that way, Finance doesn't have to come up with new money; you are simply redeploying existing resources. Cost containment should be an incentive for creativity, not a punishment for overspending. Keep your eyes on the prize.

Notes

1. "Workers Help Keep Hospital on Right TRAC, *Lima News* (May 10, 1992, pp. 1 ff).
2. Iacocca, L. *Iacocca*. New York: Bantam, 1984.
3. Taken from S. Sherman and K. Weidner, *Guidelines for Do It Groups* (Inverness, Ill.: Management House, 1991).
4. Taken from S. Sherman, *The Road to Excellence: Tools for Continuous Improvement* (Inverness, Ill.: Management House, 1992).
5. Management Engineering Services for Healthcare, "NIMC DIG Evaluation" (Madison, Wis.: University Hospital and Clinics, 1991). A private study commissioned by Northern Illinois Medical Center, McHenry, Ill.
6. Adapted from C. Sherman, *Cost Containment Audit* (Inverness, Ill.: Management House, 1986).

6

A Streamlined
Management System

There's your way, there's my way, and there's the right way.
— First-line supervisor

Organizations are directed by management, but in hospitals this is not done through systems as much as by hierarchical review and overcontrol, an inefficient approach that needs a big dose of streamlining. In this chapter, we'll see how the New American Hospital does this by using a system of management. Part of this system is a radical restructuring of how meetings are managed, the arena in which much of the manager's work has to be done. Additionally, streamlining the management system means that utilization of people is optimized; the policy, procedures, practices, and paperwork are simplified; and avenues are opened up to ensure that selling proposals and managing conflict are made easier.

A New System of Management

All organizations are run by systems — financial, data processing, and work systems. A system is a deliberately thought-out approach to best accomplish a task with the minimum amount of lost time and effort. Systems improve quality, make work easier, and increase control of the business, but many organizations do not have a management system. When management teams lack a shared system of managing, meetings don't start on time, objectives aren't set or met, and executives feel a genuine need to review too many lower-level decisions. A management system deals with the core of activities necessary for a manager to succeed, not only in work attainment, but in the political realm that organizational living represents. At one level, such a system is a series of procedures, forms, checklists, and guidelines. At a deeper level, however, it is the essence of managerial performance. Installing a management system is the best way to get work done, satisfy the boss, and turn people loose.

In the absence of being taught a specific operational approach to managing, most managers pick up the behaviors and approaches of their immediate superiors. This hit-or-miss approach often produces bad decision making, inappropriate team behavior, and collisions with political barriers.

Why is a management system needed? Organizations that have not defined proper managerial practice leave themselves open to a number of problems:

- Too much variance in management style, leading to conflict and an absence of team behavior
- Unattended responsibility areas that are ignored because of managerial drift
- Lack of team discipline and professionalism, with symptoms like go-nowhere meetings and missed deadlines
- Lack of pride, poor service attitudes, and lack of team cooperation
- Stagnant productivity, profitability, and quality

What should the system include? Specific elements of the management system that directly affect organizational functioning should:

- Specify each department's Customers and suppliers and install Customer-driven operational improvement systems
- Define the organization's value system and use it to drive organizational change and set priorities
- Supply a simple, easy-to-use planned performance system (MBO) that puts in writing what each department is going to do on a quarterly basis, clarifies authority levels, and establishes a plan of action for better results (see Chapter Five for a fuller discussion of this tool)

- Implement a work-gating procedure that selects what work will be done, focuses each department on its KRAs, and systematically identifies, minimizes, or eliminates marginal or useless work
- Supply protocols for managing change and selling proposals to make change less traumatic and easier to implement
- Release motivation by individualized work assignments and performance planning
- Deal with managing problem people by either rehabilitation or termination
- Develop constructive conflict management with a step-by-step set of procedural prescriptions
- Install procedures for effective meeting management and control
- Install effective managerial time practices, such as a Key Results Hour, which is an hour set aside every day for managers to work on a KRA problem
- Establish clear approaches to meaningful communication through Communication Centers and Associate work teams, not more newsletters
- Provide project management, work-flow diagrams, and other tools of continuous improvement and the management trade
- Specify appropriate expectations about leadership style and behavior, showing what has to be done to lead people toward work objectives
- Detail productive approaches to task-force management and the use of small-group dynamics

In my work, the written version of such a system includes specific guidelines, forms, and checklists. This represents an ideal training tool for new managers, a condensed version of what works best in management. After clarifying these things in writing, the next stage is to start making changes in the team's practices in the real world of day-to-day managing.

Meetings, Meetings, Meetings!

The true power arenas of an organization's political life are meetings. If they can be turned into dynamic, aggressive, problem-solving groups, then all the other streamlining the organization needs may come into being. Make meetings the first target in streamlining; from them will come all the other aspects of organizational excellence.

Run Meetings Right or Not at All

The ineffective manager works to create an organizational chart. The effective manager worries more about getting organized. And the true management master knows how to run meetings. Meetings consume an unbelievable amount of time and effort, particularly among managers.

One hospital president informed his management department head that meetings would start on time. He was so serious about it that at the appointed hour the door was locked. The frustrated knocking of late managers was greeted by a cacophony of laughter from the other side of the door. Their teammates were marching on! It was the last time anybody was late to a meeting!

To set the proper tone and pace in the organization, immediately move to a set of meeting management guidelines. Consider which of these items make sense in terms of improving your meetings:

- Don't have a meeting if the decision can be delegated, handled by conference call, or consolidated with another meeting, or if it is simply unnecessary.
- Don't go to meetings when a subordinate can represent you. Attend only for the time your presence is needed.
- Limit the meeting size to the minimum number of participants necessary. Group dynamics studies suggest that a group size of five to nine is optimal for most purposes. If you can reduce that number and still keep the flow going, do so. Groups of ten or more are seldom productive.

- Limit the meeting and the agenda. Set a time limit for items under discussion. Schedule meetings no earlier than the late morning in order not to interfere with Key Results Hour; the afternoon is even better. End meetings just before lunchtime or quitting time to assure cutoff. Try stand-up meetings; they never last more than twenty minutes!

- Distribute the agenda in advance. Refuse to meet if there is no agenda. Put the most important items at the top of the agenda so they are sure to be covered. Don't let the things that matter most be at the mercy of the things that matter least.

- Start on time. Don't wait for late attenders. People will never comply if there is no example of management discipline.

- Assign timekeeping and record-keeping responsibilities. Use a professional secretary. Follow the rule that all minutes are to be out within twenty-four to seventy-two hours. Keep notes only of action steps and decisions, not verbiage.

- Stick with the agenda and pace the meeting. Say, "The next point to be decided is . . ." Push forward for action and don't allow conversational drift; cut off unnecessary discussion. Don't permit interruptions except for emergencies.

- Restate conclusions and assignments to drive home what is to be done next.

Much of the change effort in creating the New American Hospital is driven by group process, such as task forces, committees, DIGs, and problem-solving groups. Unless management teaches the organization the creative use of groups and controls poor usage, much of the other work will be sacrificed. Management of meetings is a professional discipline, a prime way in which power is released in the organization.

Restructure Department Managers' Meetings

Department managers' meetings in the old hospital typically were one-way communication, with one person droning through a long list of announcements. The impact was stultifying, the image of management a disaster. As one new-breed executive said, describing his former boss, "It's no wonder he couldn't run the hospital. He didn't even know how to run a meeting!"

One of the arts of making change is to pick targets that have symbolic value, and restructuring the managers' meeting is a good one. Tell managers that it's their forum for discussion and problem solving. Announcements will no longer be made at the meeting but will be printed in a supervisory memo sent out in advance.

Managers select an agenda, make appropriate presentations, and solve problems. One effective approach is to break the managers up into small groups, with each group working on an issue a peer or executive has presented. Picture it — seventy managers buzzing around tables for twenty minutes, then presenting and debating results. The meeting becomes a forum for activists, not another sleep session. One team renamed their conference room the War Room, as a way of signaling that they were on the move.

One way to think of the importance of revitalizing this meeting is to imagine it as a center point that radiates an influence out into the rest of the organization. If the meeting sizzles, other meetings will too.

Evaluate Meetings for Results

To make sure that meetings produce results and managers act like professionals, require that all meetings be evaluated by each participant on a scale of 1 to 10 on a single question: Did this meeting produce results? Gather responses and calculate the average. That single number is then reported to the executive the committee chair reports to. The chair and the responsible executive meet when the rating falls below 8.

In the case of a nonfunctioning committee, executives ask chairpersons about the problem. Is the mission ill-defined? Are members no longer contributing what they could? Does the group need some help in the skills of managing meetings in order to get good results? Appropriate action is then taken.

The CEO's secretary monitors the average rating of all

committees and task forces and indicates to the CEO where problems are occurring. Knowing that the CEO is receiving these evaluations motivates everyone to move quickly on committees that aren't working! The CEO's secretary also inventories all committees. How many are there? How many people are participating? How many hours are being spent, and at what cost? Is the committees' productivity justifying their cost? Changes begin to occur: dead committees are abolished, nonparticipating members are removed, and meetings become leaner. This inventory process may lead to more coordinated scheduling, which increases room availability and keeps the enormity of the organization's meeting costs highly visible.

The Sunset Law

The value of task forces is that they carry their own death warrant—as soon as they complete their task, they go out of existence. On the other hand, committees tend to perpetuate themselves. Even though they may produce no results, committees seem to have eternal life.

In the New American Hospital, all committees operate under a sunset provision: they go out of existence at the end of the year unless their renewal can be justified. Justification from chairpersons should list the actual accomplishments and costs of the group in the last year. *We are not interested in having meetings; we are interested only in results.* A committee that can point with pride to fifteen or twenty major changes probably has good justification to continue. Don't tie up resources on go-nowhere, do-nothing groups. Their very presence retards and discourages organizational momentum.

Unfortunately, JCAHO requirements call for many committees and endless meetings, which generally don't produce enough to justify them as being productive. These regulations often prevent the attainment of results—they foster management by process rather than management by objectives. What is a better solution? One is to have meetings where everyone stands up. The chairperson asks, "Any old business?" "No." "Any new business?" "No." The meeting disbands. Nothing requires that a group sit there all day! On the other hand, if any required committee meetings generate good results, have more of them! If the committee structure is getting a lot of mileage, double the number of meetings. But if you're not getting much mileage out of them, ask "Why are we doing this?" Activity doesn't "feed the bulldog"; results do. Be ruthless with time. Drive it, but don't be driven by it.

Should Supervisors Be Powered Up?

In most hospitals, first-line supervisors are lead workers, or "working supervisors." They often have no direct budget authority, have limited power to initiate change, and don't even hire their own staff. In an organization struggling to handle massive change, a much larger role is called for. Power these people up.

New American Hospitals know that department heads don't pass along much of the information they receive to either first-line supervisors or Associates. How can these people become tuned in to what's going on? How can they move in the direction executives set if they don't know what it is?

One hospital president was asked by a supervisor whether she could attend department-head meetings as an observer. He accommodated this request, and he was pleasantly surprised to find that some of the better suggestions in the next few department-head meetings came from this supervisor. He increased the number of observers to four, and, finally, all members of first-line supervision were invited to the department-head meeting, which changed its name to management-team meeting. This in turn created other necessary changes. First, a larger meeting room had to be obtained. Second, since not all issues were pertinent to first-line supervisors, supervisors were given the choice of attending on an as-needed basis, which led to a much more flexible meeting schedule arrangement. However it's done, put first-line people directly into the live communication loop.

New Ways to Optimize People

Part of the old hospital's cultural legacy is that it created a mindset that rejected the notion of a classless hospital work society.

Emphasis on status and rank resulted in a poor power distribution with too much held at the top and a tremendous insufficiency at operating levels. This problem must be addressed in order to bring about a reenergized organization. One way to start is with areas that have the least power, but much to offer the cause of organizational renewal.

Power Up Low-Powered Departments

Unfortunately, a low-status, lower-power image applies to such large groups as the housekeeping staff and dietary, maintenance, and other nonpatient care areas — all essential members of the team. It doesn't matter how good cardiac surgery is if nobody picks up the garbage.

One way in which a low-powered department became a leader in the organization was shared with me recently by a new-breed executive. He informed the organization that Housekeeping had been appointed official standard bearer of the excellence renewal effort. He'd asked the housekeepers whether they were willing to set cleanliness standards so high that they would become an example to the rest of the organization. He challenged them to make the organization live up to their professionalism. Their response was tremendous. Each member of the department wore an emblem of a torch, for they were Keepers of the Flame.

Making this group the example of excellence for the rest of the organization was wise because they interacted with every department. If the people who represent Housekeeping perform at superior levels, their example shames all departments that perform at lower levels. This approach represents an excellent way to symbolically lead change, by taking a lower-status unit and making it a leader. That contrary spin is very useful in showing how we must reverse the way we're doing things.

Put Associates on Management Committees

Standing management committees and task forces need to include Associates. This isn't a bid for *equality* as much as it is an appeal for decision-making *quality*. The problem of organizational renewal isn't that Associates can't figure out what needs to be done, but that managers don't allow them to make their contribution. Typically, Associates suggest ways in which changes ought to be made, and managers immediately say, "Well, the reason it can't be done is . . ." Instead of listening to the suggestion for change, they tune out. Test this for yourself by sitting in on a meeting of managers and Associates to see whether all opinions are fully and evenly respected around the table.

Managers should educate Associates; this helps Associates sharpen the focus of their suggestions. A transition period is required to help both sides understand that each has information and knowledge the other does not. It is the successful melding of these two groups that represents hope for the organization.

As James Lincoln, founder of the Lincoln Electric Company and one of the geniuses of American management, noted in 1910:

- The progress in industry so far stems from the developed potentialities of managers. Wage earners, who because of their greater numbers have far greater potential, are overlooked. Here is where the manager must look for his greatest progress.
- The manager is dealing with expert workers far more skillful. While you can boss these experts around in the usual lofty way, their eager cooperation will not be won.
- Do unto others as you would have them do unto you. This is not just a Sunday school ideal, but a proper labor-management policy.
- If a manager [understood the reality that workers encounter], he would soon understand the real problem of management.[1]

Empower Management Horizontally

A common old hospital approach had interdepartmental problems flowing up the chain of command to a vice president, who
communicated with peers and then down that chain of command to other departments. This communication up and down
the ladder is a waste of time; it distorts whatever truth there was
to the problem to begin with and creates animosity at the
working level.

    The new management culture requires direct problem
solving between departments without line oversight. Under this
approach, a vice president whose manager reports a problem
with another department says, "Don't come to me with this. Go
to that person and solve it yourself." The only time an executive
should be involved in these squabbles and operating problems
is when the other department refuses to cooperate. This removes executives from small operational problems that waste
their time. Executives' involvement in the department head's job
is a clear sign that they don't understand their role. The payoff
for the new approach comes in greater management strength
and team spirit.

    Task forces allow managers to work horizontally across
departments and can be a primary change mechanism. But in
order for task forces to have adequate power, they must have
implementation authority on projects that affect more than the
participants' own areas. When a task force deals with problems
within a department or between departments, and all parties
that are affected are represented, the task force should be allowed to have decision-making authority that is subject to management veto only if decisions go seriously awry.

Use Rotation to Break Management Dependency

Hospital organizations present the twin problems of too much
hierarchical authority and too much departmental separation.
In turn, this creates dependency on the management structure—not sure of what to do, people wind up running to authorities. When staff people defer nearly all decisions to execu-

tives, they never grow past the point of reporting problems, always reporting the bad news but never having a solution to offer.

A number of New American Hospitals have successfully experimented with rotating middle and upper managers to departments where they do not have greater technical knowledge than the staff. This grows human talent in two ways:

1. The manager must change her leadership style to one of consultation. A manager in that situation has to say to her new staff, "I'm not the expert here, you are. I want you to help me. I want you to recommend what you think needs to be done. I want you to join me in making the decision, or make it yourself."
2. The staff is now in a position where they must bail this poor person out. In the process, they're forced to make recommendations and decisions, discovering their strength. Over time, the organization creates greater in-depth talent across its many departments.

When rotated managers move back to their original areas, they have a much better understanding of the work of the other department. They have been broadened in their view of the business and have lost much of their parochial view of the importance of their own specialty. Not only is this an effective integrating device for the organization and a builder of lower-level talent, but it also forces a management style compatible with the New American Hospital.

A counterargument is that one has to be a specialist in a field in order to supervise the people in that field. However, there are often fewer real limits than one might assume, and a number of hospitals have decided that it can be done, in at least some areas. For example, a head nurse in one specialty can assume head nurse duties in another specialty, even though she may be dependent on her staff to help with specifics.

Generally, executive transfers to other areas are not a

problem. Presidents report that this is an effective way to neutralize and educate resistant executives. As a freer situation is created for middle managers, the vice president depends on them more and more. Executive rotation is a sure way to gain some running room for middle managers. The objective is to break dependency on higher-ups and create greater confidence in taking both independent and interdependent action.

Simplifying the Four P's

The four P's of organization management are policy, procedures, practices, and paperwork. Although they're meant to be helpful in getting things done, they often wind up strangling the organization with solutions that don't fit.

Find a policy to kill. One executive found that the absenteeism policy was particularly hated by both managers and Associates. With as many managers as he could quickly find, he led a parade down to the cafeteria. Holding the policy in the air, he asked the Associates what they thought of it. They booed. He said, "What should I do with this policy?" "Burn it," came the response, whereupon he set a match to it! Send the message: policy does not control us; policy must serve us.

The skillful executive shows the management team that bureaucratic red tape strangles all their good efforts. Policies, born of a logical thought process, always lead to an illogical conclusion when they are applied to later situations. As a target for destruction, policies represent one of the greatest blockages to those managers who want to join with executives in changing things. Therefore, executive action against policy constraints encourages managers to make a contribution.

Organizational structures put a number of impeding roadblocks in the way of managerial action. A good starting point in thinking about how the organization ought to be structured is to ask managers to report the kinds of problems they have as they try to move change through the system. Make it a goal to reduce by 50 percent the number of formal controls that weigh the organization down. But don't limit the attack to policy only. The statement "That's just the way we do things here" needs to be challenged. Remember the goal: make it easier for people to get their jobs done.

If you can't get people excited about simplifying the system, try making a game out of it. One president introduced Bob's Bounties. He offered $1,000 for any committee that would vote itself out of existence, $500 if they could cut their meeting times in half, $200 for any form that could be killed off entirely, and $100 for any two forms that could be combined. The offer was good for thirty days. He spent $25,000 and estimates a first-year net savings to the organization of $1,000,000!

Simplify Policy, Reduce Approvals, and Free Budgets

Set forth guidelines that limit policies to one page, and require escape clauses that allow for managerial flexibility and judgment. Never accept policies that are just rules written for people who don't think for themselves. One of the best rules to increase communication speed is to reduce the number of approvals required to hire people, purchase equipment, and make other decisions. If a decision requires more than the sponsoring manager's signature and one level of review, it's time to ask why.

Old hospitals unnecessarily restrict budget authorities; some managers don't even have them. The New American Hospital provides monthly budgetary information to all managers. Spending authority on expense items is usually $1,000 or higher, and countersignatures are slashed. If items are approved at budget time, they don't have to be resubmitted for a second approval later. Instead of chasing down paper, the New American Hospital manager is running down problems. Budgeting freedom increases management speed, and speed is the essence of victory.

Executives still retain oversight control because managers have to stay within the budget. Spell out clearly to managers that they are being given the responsibility *and* the authority. Also let them know that there will be negative consequences if they do not handle the responsibility correctly. Your managers will not let you down.

Refine, Combine, and Discard Paper

People who study the flow of paper and work within institutions find that about 30 percent of the paperwork is completely unnecessary, and the chance that any piece of paper will ever be retrieved from a file is 5 percent. Many hospitals often require the same information to be filled in more than once, as when a patient moves from one department to another. This waste must be streamlined and costs little to do except for time. We frequently think we don't have time to fix system inefficiencies; instead we spend more time living with them than it would take to fix them. There's never time to do it right, but there's always time to do it over.

For some perverse reason, people love to design forms. These badly designed, handmade, fifth-generation, endlessly copied forms wind up creating a paper storm. Form-design software packages are useful in refining both the appearance and function of the transmitting document. Part of excellence in managing is doing what we do with some style and grace. Homemade paper forms communicate an amateurish attitude and lack polish, especially when they are seen by Customers who are used to dealing with better-run organizations.

It is important to combine forms, or to have task forces study the real flow of the work. Focus initially on simple tasks, then on high-impact and volume processes. A total system review, while logical, isn't always easy or timely to pull off. Get started on pieces of it; when they are finally put into a total system review, it will be in better shape. The goal is to reduce the paper blizzard, starting with the paper afflicting management. Attack early on the phenomenon in which managers memo everybody. Go to the one-page memo. Under no circumstances allow conflict or accusations to be put on paper.

Selling Ideas More Easily

Streamlining the system isn't just a matter of cleaning up the clutter. Managers need to know how to put new pieces into the system, sell proposals, and overcome resistance.

Selling Proposals with Structured Guidelines

Streamlining means selling a lot of new ideas. Managers report that selling an idea in the old hospital was like being a salmon going up-river, a battle all the way. While the New American Hospital provides a much more receptive selling environment for ideas, managers still need to learn the skill of selling proposals. One answer has been to set up guidelines that list the criteria executives will be looking for. A standard format for organizing the proposal can also be helpful. Typically, executives like to see data in certain display formats; this can be incorporated into the organization's management system. Agreement on the format and package by the top executive team takes some of the risk out of the selling process for managers and gives new ideas a higher survival rate. Remember, we're trying to create an organization where selling ideas becomes a smooth process, and these are skills that managers must learn. Spell out for managers how to sell their ideas so that everyone may win. Exhibit 6.1 gives an example of how this was done at one hospital.

One absolute change requirement is to consult all affected departments in advance of the proposal's implementation. Nursing cannot make any changes that affect another department if that department has not been consulted. The building czar whose staff show up without the department manager knowing anything about it will be hung at sunrise! This behavior reflects a lack of team thinking and is usually a bad solution to boot. It's amateur management at its worst and must be forbidden.

As a corollary, any program that is going to require a fair amount of time or work has to be allowed sufficient time to be put into practice. The staff department that requires a change within thirty days, but that has not consulted the affected departments about what is realistic given their existing workload, has just lost points in the informal world.

Teaching Change by Making Examples

In the 1700s, the British admiralty gave a standing guideline to captains of the fleet: find someone insubordinate enough to

Exhibit 6.1. A Short Test of Proposal Worthiness.

The following checklist of items has been found to be useful to make sure that your idea is in good enough shape to be presented.

1. Does it fit the values statement of our organization?
    *   Excellence
    *   Respect
    *   Service
2. Does it fit with the seven Key Result Areas expected in your job? If it doesn't, your boss might ask why you're involved with it at all! Does this idea have anything to do with:
    *   Customer satisfaction
    *   Quality
    *   People growth
    *   Organizational climate
    *   Innovation
    *   Productivity
    *   Economics
3. Is it something that a significant portion of your Customers want you to do, something that they need? Or is it only a pet project or something you think the public wants with no basis for that opinion?
4. Does it provide any competitive advantage? Is it important to maintain or increase our market share?
5. What are the economic or financial considerations? Does it generate enough revenue or reduce other costs enough to pay its own way?
6. Will other projects or services have to be delayed or not done if this proposal is implemented?
7. How important is it to the long-term future of the organization? Is it just a passing fad that will not be significant for an extended period of time?
8. Does the project meet the test of the major emphases that your executives are interested in today, such as increased market share and profitability?

---

flog or hang and do it before the crew. This was meant to be instructional to the crew, showing that the captain's word was law.

The New American Hospital does not want a repressive or fearful tone. But executives should be on the lookout for "Stalinists," those who resist change and are maintaining the old system, refusing to join in its evolution, and sandbagging the future. They do not want the status quo of the old system disrupted, and they misuse their power by stalling. They jealously guard the rigid power centers that must be jettisoned in any effort to create a free-flowing system. Although their numbers are not great, they present a barrier that needs to be dealt with.

One New American Hospital president had just started his change program when one of his department managers decided to ignore his authority by failing to live up to a change requirement. The manager had always been a problem and had not contributed for years. The president called him into his office. With absolute glee, he informed the manager that he had been looking for an opportunity to set an example of how he would deal with resistance to change in the system. Rubbing his hands with joy, he said, "Ralph, you're it!" Ralph was gone by the end of that day.

Studies of successful change executives show that replacement of a few personnel is one of the best strategies to pursue in making your views known. Who is supported, and who isn't, tells people all they need to know about whether the desire to change the system is serious. The flip side of the coin is even more true. Find folks struggling to make improvements in the system and make heroes out of them. All kinds of good things should happen to those who take on the status quo and turn it into a great future.

Turn Conflict into Creative Energy

The old hospital saw conflict as bad, something to be avoided. The New American Hospital knows that conflict is energy, but it needs to be converted from a destructive force to a constructive one. None of us could live in the presence of atomic radiation, but when it is converted to electrical energy it becomes useful. How can an organization use the human frustration that results when achievement is blocked, or the energy spent butting heads when people pursue their own agendas against the flow of others? How do we make the conversion?

An early assignment I recommend is for managers to work in departments with which they have a high degree of interaction. Managerial swaps may involve doing menial chores within a department as well as getting to know the people and what they need. These swaps are followed by others between key staff members. Over time, as this works through the departments, even new Associates are assigned to work for a short period of time as part of their orientation. Just getting to know people and understanding what they do can dramatically lower the amount of conflict in the organization.

Make Conflict Manageable by Defining Procedures

When conflict or working problems occur between depart-ments that have been following a swapping procedure, much less arguing ensues because a relationship of personal trust has been established. A problem-solving swap is worked out, with appropriate staff sent to the other department or shift to study the problem from its point of view. The visiting representative approaches the problem with this question, "What is it that *we* could do to make things better?" That question quickly creates a team discussion of how to improve the situation.

The New American Hospital knows that conflict is toxic waste that can quickly poison relationships. Conflict must be managed, not tolerated or ignored. Procedures like the problem-solving swap need to be made part of the formal man-agement system. Other conflict-management elements include required direct communication between conflicting parties without informing their bosses, presentation of gifts to denote respect, time deadlines to resolve the problem, and notes to the file of anyone who refuses to follow the new procedures. Conflict must be managed in order to avoid damaging people and relationships.

Aid Innovation by Using Constructive Confrontation

One New American Hospital practice that raises eyebrows is the use of conflict as a positive source of constructive change. Con-structive confrontation is an important new management prin-ciple that says that facts and expertise should decide issues, not rank, power, or status. When decisions are made based on executive opinion, and the truth known by others is discounted, the organization's business interests are placed in jeopardy.

Constructive confrontation gives everyone permission to continue raising issues up to the point when a decision is made, even if they are opposed by ranking executives. This permission forbids executives to punish others who are attempting to "save the bacon." James Burke, CEO of Johnson & Johnson, reports that this concept has been an important contribution to their management culture, and that even the youngest employees, given the freedom to debate fiercely, are often more right than the most dignified senior executive. In the end, everybody wins. Says Burke:

> We have some very tough meetings, very open and often emotion-filled. It is a style of management I have always encouraged. By putting a lot of contention into our system we get better results. Certainly it makes us more honest with each other. I don't think it bruises people to argue and debate. You'd be surprised how easy some of our young people find it to politely say, "You know, you're wrong. . . . You don't have the facts. . . I do. . . and here's the evidence to prove it." You then begin to get into the kind of debate that helps to make us all think better and helps us to reach a more satisfactory solution. This openness also makes people understand that we try hard to be fair. Anyone with the right answer, no matter who he or she is, is going to be respected. In recent years contention has become a part of our management culture, and as long as it remains constructive I encourage it. To suppress talented people from speaking their minds is to deny yourself your most important resource — ideas![2]

Obviously, the proponent of a particular viewpoint must know the facts, must be willing to do the homework required, and must be prepared to argue for the cause. This element of the New American Hospital's management culture requires executives to remain open and be patient while others make their case. Give it a try.

A Test: Can People Work Freely, Efficiently, and Cooperatively?

The purpose of streamlining the system is to allow people to get their work done in the easiest possible way, at the least possible cost, and in a way that builds cooperative relationships. If the ideas presented in this chapter do not seem attractive, then ask whether your people work freely, efficiently, and cooperatively. The experience of many New American Hospitals is that making streamlining changes like those in this chapter skyrockets the ability of people to work more easily and effectively.

Notes

1.   Harvard Business School Case Services, *The Lincoln Electric Company* (Boston, Mass.: Harvard Business School, 1975), pp. 19–20.
2.   J. Burke quoted in T. R. Horton, *What Works for Me: 16 CEOs Talk About Their Careers and Commitments* (New York: Random House, 1986).

7

Optimizing Organizational Structure

> Our most melancholy thoughts about organization almost
> always concern the classic bureaucracy — a thing of divisions,
> branches, bureaus and departments, through which flow
> rivers of memoranda. In terms of status, it is a pyramid, and
> only a few at the top have the faintest idea what the whole
> organization is about.
>
> —John W. Gardner,
> *Self-Renewal*[1]

Revitalization and renewal are often hampered by the formal
organizational patterns existing in the old hospital. Healing the
hospital means *ridding the organization of the breaks and fractures*
that prevent humans from knitting together in productive enterprise. *Structural reenergizing* can be started by making a number
of simple and easy changes. More difficult is the next wave of
changes that focus on *structuring the organization to better serve
Customers.* Against the things that can easily be done with the old
structure is set the picture of *structures found in the New American
Hospital.* Finally, the chapter looks again at some *organizational
fundamentals* that serve as a useful checklist for the organization
to meet proper design specifications.

Healing the Fractured Hospital

The old hospital is sick and presents many symptoms of its
illness. To the extent that it has morale problems, its heart is sick.
To the extent that it can't generate ideas and implement innovations, its brain is sick. To the degree that it doesn't accept change,
it can't digest risks. And when it can't freely move and can't lift its

The opening quotation of this page is reprinted by permission of Sterling
Lord Literistic, Inc. Copyright © 1963 by John W. Gardner.

load, something is fractured in the bones that we call organization. Organizational structure can be thought of as the skeleton upon which many of the hospital's systems function. Today that skeleton is fractured, osteoporotic, and weak. It needs fundamental rehabilitation or replacement.

The typical hospital is well organized vertically, but poorly organized horizontally. Old hospitals are organized around functional specialties and are referred to as *functional organizations*. They lump specialists together so that nurses, laboratory personnel, and housekeepers each have separate enclaves and identified turfs. This creates a segregated society that is clearly visible in the cafeteria, where the white uniforms, green uniforms, and gray uniforms all dine separately.

Segregated Organizations Have Inherent Problems

Functional organizations are dysfunctional. Like any segregated society, they pay a price. Following are some characteristic problems within functional organizations:

- Segregation is caused by the organizational structure itself. Departments and their divisions, levels, and layers act to produce distrust, paranoia, "turfism," and power plays.
- Isolating specialists based on their knowledge means isolating them in their ignorance. Progress is held up as much by nurses who don't understand finance as it is by staff in Central Supply who don't see the reality of bedside care. All parties are innocently wrong, but wrong nonetheless.
- The chain of command unintentionally becomes the chain of communication. By restraining and slowing communication, the chain of command produces lethargy and inertia.
- Decisions tend to funnel up to the apex of the hierarchy. In a rapidly changing environment more and more decisions must move up to a few decision makers, a bottleneck that means too little change processed per unit of time.
- Layered organizations are poor at communicating accurately and in a timely way, with a resulting fall-off in decision-making speed and accuracy.

- Quality problems are inherent when the left hand doesn't know what the right hand is doing. Departmental isolation is a repeating theme in quality errors.
- Those who are considered to be lower-status feel a loss of morale and job zest and a passive dependency. Turnover and unionization are on the horizon for too many hospitals as a result.
- Customer irritation and anger result when problems are left untended. As they pile up, Customers wonder, "Who's on first?"

Structural Change Is Not Organizational Change

A common executive mistake is overestimating the amount of organizational change that can be achieved by changing the organizational structure. It is far more important to restructure working relationships than to redraw charts. Some hospitals focus too much on playing with the organizational chart and on who reports to whom. The goal is to create a hospital whose individual pieces operate so effectively together that its primary targets as a service organization are smoothly achieved. This may or may not require structural change. Structural changes are often called for in the hospital world and this may be a useful area to consider, but don't be fooled into seeing this as a magic pill. And don't get caught in the mindset that views the human organization as a set of lines and boxes. The best chart is whatever works for the people.

Getting Started with Structural Change

In many cases, restructuring the organization is a no-cost variable, useful to both instigate and consolidate change. My view of structural design in the New American Hospital is that it should take place within the much larger and more important arena of organizational revitalization. The objectives of redesign in this context are to create a structure that:

- Achieves an organizational design that serves Customer needs
- Accelerates people growth and enhances team operation and morale, redistributing power and changing roles at all levels
- Overcomes the existing problems of functional segregation
- Expedites work accomplishment and has the supporting characteristics of easy communication flow, fast decision making, and ease of implementation
- Is both an outcome and a creator of renewal and eventual organizational excellence

Blur the Chain of Command

Skilled change executives say that it's often best to ignore the chart. As they begin to change the organization, they don't issue printed updates, and they pay little attention to the lines and boxes. This *intelligent inattention* to the organizational chart blurs the chain of command. Think of all the work, time, and hand-holding effort these savvy executives are saving!

Just tell people that their boss is the Customer and they should do what the Customer wants. After the initial clamor to use the chart as a crutch dies down, most people begin to think in a more relaxed fashion. For others, the lack of uncertainty creates an anxiety that puts them on their toes and opens them up to additional change. Perhaps the one change your organizational structure needs more than any other is to have people pay no attention to it! What about regulators' requirements that there be a chart? There's probably an old one somewhere in the file.

Install the First Amendment

How bad would it be if your people began to think, "I can go anywhere, talk to anybody about anything at any time, and I don't need permission"? Announce to your people that the First Amendment regarding freedom of speech and thought applies at your shop, too. It built a great nation, and it will build a great hospital. Free up the intellect, and watch greatness happen!

Unfortunately for many old hospitals, the chain of command has become the chain of communication. There ought to be a clear chain of accountability, but this concept is always a little fuzzy in a hospital where decisions should be made on the basis of who has the knowledge, not who has the title. Imposing the chain of command on communication prevents communication from taking place without approval from a higher-level authority, the kiss of death in the rapidly changing world in which hospitals now operate. People have to be able to talk to anyone they want to, any time they want to, about any issue— now! Decisions may still require chain-of-command approval, but there should be no required chain of communication.

Use the Phone Book as an Organizational Chart

In nearly all hospitals, Associates' names aren't in the phone book. Why not? Everywhere in the United States, the phone company lists everybody's name, and it helps communication. Yet, in most hospital phone books, only the managers' names and departmental references are given. This is old hospital thinking—listing only managers' names makes the book a status symbol. What nonsense!

Suppose that a new employee wants to order a lab test. She looks in the hospital phone book and finds only the manager's name. She calls, steering a piece of nonmanagement work to a manager who must interrupt his work to take the order or tell her to call someone else. This is a waste of management time, and it turns managers into telephone operators forwarding calls.

New American Hospitals include all Associates' names in white pages listed alphabetically, and in yellow pages by subject heading. In the old hospital, people keep little lists of numbers of people to call to get things done—why not just put them into a phone book?

Create New Groupings to Increase Speed

A number of changes can be made in a functionally divided organization to reduce the negative effects of segregation. Some new leaders believe that it's best to proceed gradually with organizational change, following an evolutionary course toward radical structures. At other times a more rapid course may be best. Following are two ideas that have been successful for those of the gradualist school.

Put Noncooperating Departments Under the Same Executive. Gaps that exist between departments are usually greatest between divisions. Departments reporting to different executives tend to compound their problems if the executives are squabbling. One New American Hospital president got tired of hearing of the ruckus between Nursing and Admitting. By putting them both under one executive, problems suddenly got solved! Sometimes this device can be done just long enough to solve a problem. Grouping under a common management provides proximity, an exchange of knowledge, and the same steely-eyed boss.

Consolidate Departments. One- and two-person departments are a monument to somebody's ego. Professional identity should be based on contribution, not an organizational shell. Group small departments together, if that makes sense, or attach them to a larger unit. Fewer divisional and departmental walls mean fewer barriers between people. And fewer departments, but with the same number of specialties, might make your organizational problems easier to live with. At the same time, look at the political question of how these people will be given adequate voice if they are grouped together. Simplify, simplify.

Reduce Management Levels to a Maximum of Four

Organizations with fewer levels have faster communication, faster and more accurate decision making, higher Customer satisfaction, higher productivity, and better worker morale. These findings give credence to the concept that in organizational structuring, less is more. The best kinds of organizations are those that allow people to move freely to deal with the work at hand. New American Hospitals systematically reduce the number of working levels of management to no more than four, with three being preferable: an executive layer, a middle-management (department-head) level, and first-line supervision. Any more is a waste. Get rid of all "assistant-to" positions. If the person in that position needs an assistant, you need a new manager.

A hospital is not primarily a linear, throughput system, in which a strong hierarchy is sometimes appropriate. It is highly interactive, with a lot of movement back and forth between departments, as well as vertical commands and political influence. It's not uncommon in medium-sized hospitals to find as many as six or seven layers of management. The effect of an increasingly top-heavy bureaucracy is to strangle those at lower levels and cripple their accomplishments. People struggle against the bureaucracy and exhaust themselves. Said one manager, "It's like swimming in peanut butter."

A variation on this theme are the new corporate structures being set up in some multihospital systems where corporate officers are adding staffs, imposing two or three layers on top of an already heavy field hospital organizational structure. This sows the seeds of defeat. My experience in dealing with hospitals that are part of a corporate system is that they are slower, more hamstrung, and greatly frustrated. Whatever benefits may accrue from being part of a system are to some degree offset by lack of local control. This is a direct result of increased layering, not bad people. The best approach being taken by some systems is to follow Alfred P. Sloan's dictum when he led General Motors: "Centralized policy, decentralized control." Give the people in the field their head; help them by staying out of their way.

Reduce the Number of Vice Presidents

Just as reducing the number of layers increases information flow and speed vertically, reducing the number of vice presidencies increases flow horizontally. Having fewer divisions simplifies operations. With a reduction of levels, the organization be-comes flatter. With a reduction of divisions, it becomes leaner.

Recently in an old hospital I faced an executive group with no fewer than seventeen vice presidents representing five levels among them (an executive vice president, senior vice presidents, vice presidents, associate vice presidents, and as-sistant vice presidents)! Do we really need that much help? We can run the United States with only one! The more vice presi-dents there are, the weaker the managers are. Organizational obesity starts at the top, and flabbiness at command levels never produces Olympic performance.

Reduction of executives and management levels can often occur through normal attrition, like a gradual weight loss pro-gram. In other cases it makes more sense to get it done quickly, either because there's no time to wait or because nervousness exists about when this particular shoe will drop. Do it slow or do it fast, but do it!

Restructuring for Customer Service

The organization exists to serve its primary Customer, the pa-tient. While there are other Customers such as physicians and visitors, the first and most important test of an adequate hospi-tal structural design should be whether patients are served by it.

Product Line Management

Figure 7.1 shows the four major forms of traditional organiza-tional design. Old hospitals are primarily *functional* organiza-tions, and that needs to change. No organization exists as a pure form of any of these structures, but articulating that the organi-zation needs to move away from a too-great focus on functional design leads to the question of what design concepts we wish to include.

To the extent that a hospital has active task forces that cut across departmental lines, they are involved in a *project manager* structure. Such arrangements create a dotted-line authority from the project manager to the specialists in each of the

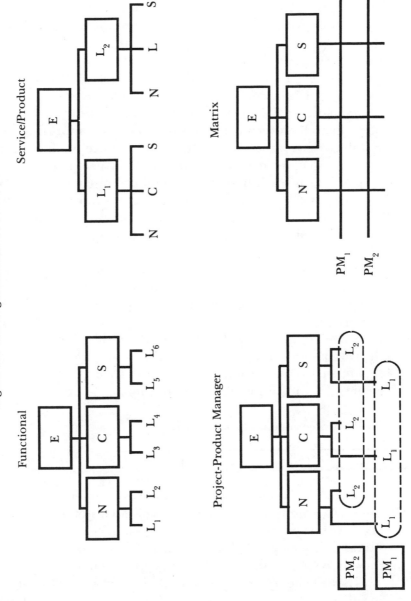

Figure 7.1. Old Organizational Structures.

functional areas. Each member of the project team has a direct-line reporting relationship to the function area's executive. The horizontal grouping is a necessary integrator to work around the segregation problem, but these arrangements are usually temporary.

Service–product line management groups all departments serving a product line, such as mothers and newborns, under a single manager. This permits easier coordination between departments; however, it also creates multiple reporting relationships that may lead to confusion. The concept is logical, but it is not useful in smaller hospitals where departments can't be divided. What often happens is a compromise effort, as when Pharmacy sets up a satellite dispensing unit on the maternity floor. A worse approach is to create a new level of manager in the unit to coordinate with all other departments.

The *matrix* as an organizational form is not applicable to hospitals. There appears to be no correlation between matrix organization and excellence in business performance. The matrix may have some applicability in organizations that are very large (in excess of one hundred thousand Associates) or where there are complex supplier relationships (like NASA and its thirty thousand suppliers). Even in these complex applications, this form has not worked very well. I strongly recommend against it for it confuses and complicates.

Fit the Structure to Customer Needs

A cardinal design rule is that form should follow function. The organizational chart and the manner in which people operate should follow the function and purposes for which the organization was created — to serve the needs of its Customers. Customers move horizontally, not vertically, through health care organizations. They may hobble down the hall or roll on gurneys, but they always move horizontally from department to department. This is the primary argument for taking a service-line approach in an organization that wants its form to follow function in providing direct service. Any attempt that can be made, either physically or on a reporting basis, to locate people where they can best serve the Customer shows form following function. It is less important to design the organizational chart to fit a service-line concept than it is to design the work flow so that the handoffs between departments are seamless and flawless as far as the Customer is concerned.

Frequently, all nursing departments are under one executive, and all laboratory and testing units are under another. Why not group all departments that have direct patient contact under a common executive? This isn't product-line management where we're concerned about horizontal reporting relationships, but rather a way to combine all departments serving patients (Nursing, Housekeeping, Dietary, and Laboratory Services) under the same executive. The functional organization remains, but the political reality is that everyone must now cooperate.

Structures in the New American Hospital

A number of novel approaches to visualizing the organization have been taken in New American Hospitals. While they are widely divergent, they all have the common characteristic of being primarily concerned with teaching the organization how to think about itself and its role, and little to do with illustrating the chain of command.

Flip Their Minds by Flipping the Chart

Figure 7.2 contrasts old and new organizational structures as pictured by one hospital president to highlight a contrarian change. On the left is the old structure; on the right is the new. Usually, publishing the organizational chart in a period of change is counterproductive: everybody worries too much about the pecking order. In this case it worked wonderfully as a tool to assist change.

Here's why visualizing the organization upside-down succeeded:

- It lowered the power image of executives and raised the power image of Associates. Executives were pictured as

Figure 7.2. Redistributed Power Organization.

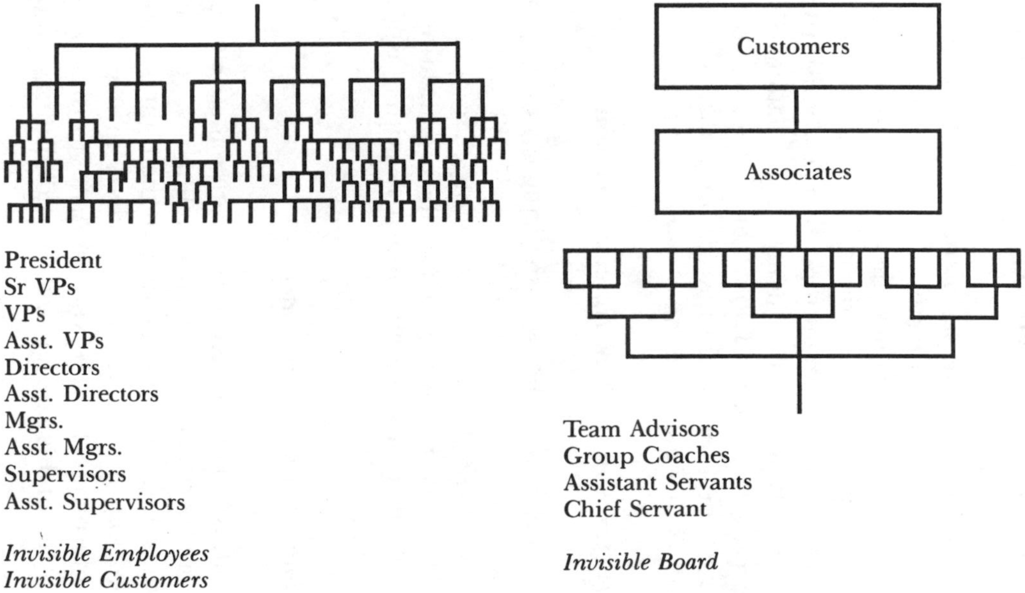

President
Sr VPs
VPs
Asst. VPs
Directors
Asst. Directors
Mgrs.
Asst. Mgrs.
Supervisors
Asst. Supervisors

Invisible Employees
Invisible Customers

Customers

Associates

Team Advisors
Group Coaches
Assistant Servants
Chief Servant

Invisible Board

working for Associates, not the other way around. Associates had no resistance to this idea!

- It immediately took away resistant energy from those executives who might have fought the concept. This is essential to good change management.
- It made clear that the Customer is boss, a focus everyone can buy into. Note: This is the only organizational chart ever seen where the Customer is even mentioned!
- Management ranks were noticeably less layered and sported the new titles they picked for themselves.
- There were markedly fewer departments and divisions.

This approach resulted in a leaner organization and affected status, roles, motivation, and attitudes, all in a positive way. It also pointed the organization toward its prime objective, Customer service. Not bad for a simple diagram!

Other New American Hospital Designs

Out of the creativity of people feeling their way on this design question have come numerous structures. Figure 7.3 shows two of them.

In example A, the cluster of dots represents the organizational chart issued by one president. Each dot represents an Associate or manager. The true organization is seen when any combination of three or eight or twenty-three dots interact to fix a problem. As a Customer goes through a hospital stay, many dots — arrayed in chains, pairs, or groups — may interact with the Customer. This concept of organization is pictured here as a sociogram. Juncture points where many lines are drawn and redrawn over a number of episodes are the true power centers of the organization. This particular visualization was appropriate for this hospital because the president wanted to keep people guessing as to how he would eventually structure various reporting relationships. He wanted to underscore that who was in charge was a lot less important than strengthening the bonds — the lines — between the people represented by the dots. This also

Figure 7.3. Other New American Hospital Designs.

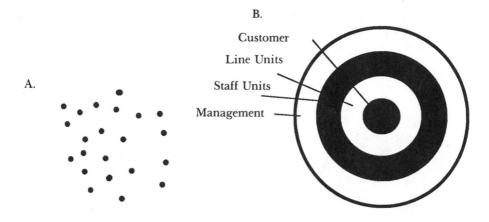

sent a message to the power-hungry that they were an equal among equals.

In example B, another hospital president sees the organization as a target, where the bull's-eye is the Customer. The entire hospital is organized around this center, with the most important departments being the line units. This means a redefinition from old hospital thinking, because staff from Housekeeping, Food Services, and the laboratory are in the patient's room and are therefore considered as much line staff as Nursing is. Staff units include Central Supply and Maintenance. This was an appropriate message for this organization, in which the president wanted to power up previously low-powered departments. He also wanted to send a message to staff groups and to management that they were there only to serve the line and, through the line units, to serve the Customer.

What's the best way to picture things in your organization? Should you publish a picture at all, or publish it in phases? What kind of impact do you want it to have? These are the appropriate questions for structural design when it is wedded to the more important questions of organizational change.

Publish Role Descriptions

Whether you publish an organizational chart or not, you should definitely publish New American Hospital role descriptions. Exhibit 7.1 can be modified, but organizations that have used it suggest limiting it to a page and posting it throughout the house.

Organizing Basics

If you've done what the New American Hospital calls for, then what follows is unnecessary. But it's hard for some executives to give up the security blanket of a good solid chart. For those who insist on muddling through with an old form structure, please read on. Even traditional forms can be made to work better if they are accompanied by many of the other themes this book represents.

What are the key principles or "rules" of organizing for work accomplishment? Keep these in mind as you wrestle with departmental and organization-wide structural problems.

Have Clearly Focused Organizing Objectives

Hospitals benefit when managers sit back and ask some basic questions: Where are we going? What do we want to achieve? What are our objectives and goals? It is not uncommon for the failing organization to forget its original mission and the reasons for its very existence—for example, when hospitals formed to serve the poor now turn away the indigent.

Remember to stay Customer-focused. Define the organization's Customers and markets. The primary reality, even before questions of finance, is that organizations exist not to serve themselves, but to serve the needs of their market. Although this seemingly is an obvious point, it is often overlooked. Ask: What does the Customer want and need? How can we best serve the

The "Organizing Basics" portion of this chapter is reprinted from V. C. Sherman, "Organizing for Strength," *Personal Journal* (Costa Mesa, Calif.: July 1979).

Exhibit 7.1. New American Hospital Role Descriptions.

AT OUR NEW AMERICAN HOSPITAL . . .
Customers Are Kings and Queens
Our success depends on excellent care for the Customer. Our job is to meet
their needs. We have many different Customers: patients, visitors, physicians,
other departments, and Associates. If we can't solve a Customer's problem,
ask why, and suggest changes to our system. Customers have most of the ideas
that will improve our system, and their evaluation of our performance is the
basis for our pay. They honor us by bringing us difficult problems. It is a
privilege to serve them.

Associates Are a Team and Have Power to Act
Associates are the most important people on the payroll. Their care, skills,
and experience combine to reach our one standard of performance—excellence in all that we do. Associates have the freedom to challenge policy and to
continuously improve the way we do things. They are represented in all
management groups and communication channels. They chair a majority of
Do It Groups and Customer Satisfaction Councils. Whatever they need to get
the job done is what the organization must do its best to fulfill. Associates are
a team, not just a group of individuals. They are a family where each helps the
other. They are the organization. What the hospital will be grows out of what
they are. They live the values at all times and focus on KRA targets.

Management Advises and Coordinates Operations
Team advisers and coaches work for their Associates and are accountable for
whatever support Associates need. They stay in close touch with Associates
and Customers to understand the needs that may exist, but do not impede
the work of Associates. Their role is to advise, teach, coach, and recognize in
order to build the team. At all times, they lead by example and protect their
departmental team and those working in other departments. Managers make
decisions on-site and work with other members of management to solve all in-
house operating problems. They involve executives only in rare instances. If
managers are not sure what to do, they ask Associates or Customers. They live
the values at all times and focus on KRA targets.

Executives Plan, Find Resources, and Recognize Performance
Assistant Servants and the Chief Servant are here only to help others get their
jobs done in serving the Customer. Their job is to get the organization ready
for change and to find ways to come up with resources for all the things we
need. They are responsible for developing new ways to recognize and reward
everyone for excellence of achievement. Executives do not get involved in
operating problems except as Associates or managers request. They are here
to protect the organizational family in the way a loving parent would.
Executives are here to push things along, to make sure that the conditions of
freedom and information are present, and to remove obstacles affecting our
future. They live the values at all times and focus on KRA targets.

Customer's interests? When these basic questions can be answered in some detail, then an examination of the organization's structure is in order.

Finally, ask: What are the key success factors (KSFs) for this kind of business? The New American Hospital knows that some of its KSFs are speed of service, high efficiency, fail-safe quality, and mastery of cultural change. If they are necessary for the hospital to be successful, what kind of organizational structure will help to deliver them? Ask the questions first. Then, and only then, are you ready to consider how to organize.

Certain structural basics have been found useful when thinking through how to organize:

- *Don't overorganize.* Don't divide things up to the point where nobody's job is fun. Keep the organization as compact as possible, without too many layers or too much middle spread.
- *Watch the span of control.* Generally, a manager should have no more than seven people reporting directly to him or her. On the other hand, some organizations deliberately violate this rule, since they find that it forces downward delegation. If you want everybody to report to you, is it because you think that people can't be trusted?
- *Specify a chain of command.* The line of control from top to bottom must be clearly specified for every department. Who is in charge, as well as his or her superior, should be answerable for every unit.
- *Emphasize unity of command.* Each employee in the organization should receive orders from, and report to, only one supervisor (a principle that is cheerfully forgotten in service-line organizations). Split or overlapping authority can be a cause of organizational shipwreck.
- *Specify line thrust.* Don't allow battles between line and staff units, and don't let line managers lord it over the staff units. Clearly spell out which units are most directly involved with the market or with meeting primary objectives. Not all units are created equal, and an organization is not a democracy.
- *Provide for staff controls.* Staff units should be involved in most

major policy decisions. While they may not issue orders to the line organization, they should exercise controls through policy channels and action review.

- *Force decision making downward.* This is done simply by reducing the number of layers and increasing the span of control within acceptable limits. Decisions made closer to the scene of the action are usually better.

- *Watch status symbols.* Appropriate status rewards should accompany elevation in the hierarchy, or what's a heaven for? But make sure that this isn't overdone. Studies of supervisory effectiveness indicate that too much separation between the leader and the led is counterproductive.

- *Consolidate and trim.* Where possible, lump units together to avoid specialization and increase the possibility of synergy. Trim excess fat, eliminate units that once served an important purpose but no longer do, or redefine them with a new mission.

Restore People Primacy

People existed before organizations—they are real. Organizations are an intellectual construct—they are artificial. Organizational charts are not holy and unchangeable. Don't become so preoccupied with drawing little boxes and lines that you begin to think of the diagram as having any inherent value. The people you place in the boxes are the ones who make the corporate plane fly. What works for them? Some believe that a structure should be laid out first and people should then be crammed into it, like so many round pegs in square holes. One suggestion is that you examine the strengths of your key people and then organize the structure around them. Just as a tailor-made suit looks better than one off the rack, so the tailor-made organization will be a better fit for the people who have to wear it.

Remember to protect the informal organization. Where possible, play into the group alliances, professional cliques, and special interests. Formal organization tends to be stronger when it follows informal relationships and interaction patterns. The organizational chart is two-dimensional, but the human organization is three-dimensional. Some managers get all tied up in their emotions when people circumvent official channels. If workers are doing the job, don't worry about it.

Make upward communication happen. It won't, unless management makes it happen. Organizational layering, with its corresponding status and authority intimidation, tends to screen out nearly all of the real information about what's happening at the operating levels. In essence, this means that conditions occurring on the battlefield need to be reported directly to command headquarters by forward observers. Generals are advised to talk directly with privates and to remember that the organizational chart they so lovingly designed works against them. Don't let your staff isolate you from the people.

Note

1. J. W. Gardner, *Self-Renewal: The Individual and the Innovative Society* (New York: HarperCollins, 1964), p. 82.

Part Three

SUCCEEDING IN
ORGANIZATIONAL RENEWAL

8

Leading the Transition

> As an old system cracks, the faceless bureaucrat-managers
> who run it are blown away by a guerrilla army of risk-
> taking investors, promoters, organizers, and managers,
> many of them antibureaucratic individualists, all of them
> skilled at either acquiring knowledge or controlling its
> dissemination. . . .
> For the task of restructuring companies and whole indus-
> tries to survive in the super-symbolic economy is not a job for
> nit-picking, face saving, bean-counting bureaucrats. It is, in
> fact, a job for individualists, radicals, gut-fighters, even eccen-
> trics—business commandos, as it were, ready to storm any
> beach to seize power.
>
> —Alvin Toffler
> *Power Shift*[1]

The New American Hospital requires a new type of executive
leader. The work of that leader is to create the kind of organizational climate that allows successful rebirth. In turn, a new form
of managerial leadership is required, as well as a new mission for
managers as they take on the real work of transforming the
organization at the essential level of daily operations. The chapter also looks at the kind of leadership symbols and behavior
that will be helpful in managing the new organization; finally,
the chapter discusses the career management issues of selecting
winners, developing them to reach their potential, and removing them if they can't perform. Now, more than ever, we see how
essential the work of leadership has become to the future of
health care.

The New Leader

Both executive and managerial roles in the New American Hospital have to undergo major restructuring. Unless they do, it is impossible for all of the other needed changes to follow. Restructuring not only means changing the concept of the job but changing the systems, operating procedures, and formal authorities that spell out how things are done. Unless the organization's executives and managers can pull off the changes described in this chapter, the rest of the change agenda cannot be achieved.

Does the CEO Have Horsepower and Vision?

Does your hospital's president have the horsepower necessary to pull off a major organization development effort? The president doesn't have to be Lee Iacocca or Ross Perot, but there needs to be enough toughness, emotion, vision, and dissatisfaction with the status quo to drive the system through its change processes. Has the CEO got the oomph to get the job done?

Organizational change requires a tremendous sense of direction and motivation to change. In the early stages, most of this energy and drive has to come from the CEO. If that person doesn't have what it takes, organization development becomes an academic exercise.

Heal Executive Schisms to Create Top Unity

If there are interpersonal blockages in the executive team, the individuals involved need to work out those differences and literally shake hands in front of their peers. While this is an uncomfortable experience for some, it removes the wedges between key players. Burying hatchets, smoking peace pipes, and building bridges at the top are necessary for a new beginning.

At one conference, the corporate system's CEO and the hospital's CEO had been instructed to sit side by side with each other. On the first day of the conference, they refused and sat on opposite sides from each other in the horseshoe. Their people,

seeing the usual split in their top leadership, insisted on maintaining all of their old fixed positions and lined up on opposite
sides of the room. As the conference leader, I called the two
together and told them that if they were not prepared to shake
hands and start functioning like a team, I was leaving. That
forced a negotiation. Sometimes positive desire is enough to
bring about team unity. Sometimes you must knock heads together and create a situation in which disunity brings with it too
high a price.

Go to the Mountain

As change agents, we have often found value in taking the
executive team to a conference center for a thorough discussion
on what the New American Hospital represents and to discuss
the operating changes called for in undertaking such a project.
It's essential to open a detailed and heartfelt discussion with
those who are taking the risk of making major organizational
change. Invariably, differences emerge between executives concerning the need for change, past communication chasms, and
political baggage. This old business has to be dealt with quickly
if the effort is to move forward.

At the meeting the team needs to understand what the
change model will look like, but even more important is the
need to unfreeze old attitudes. Skillful executives are not afraid
of the group dynamics that are unleashed in these sessions. This
is an opportunity to vent, to listen to submerged thinking, to
confront the issues that have been tiptoed around in the past,
and to begin purging the team of false thinking. Obstructionists
soon make themselves known, and a healthy opportunity is
created to "get it together." The building of consensus is essential. Unless this can be done at the executive level, the change
effort will fail or be severely damaged.

The Executive as Listener, Servant, Cheerleader, and Visionary

In the old definition, the executive was the speaker from Mount
Olympus, the order giver, the superior, the boss, and the power

center. In the New American Hospital, the executive's job becomes that of listener, facilitator, integrator, servant, and vision-
ary. This strongly suggests some title changes.

One definition of the executive's job is that of the vision-
ary, the dream speaker, who sketches what the future looks like
on the distant horizon, and who continually spreads this vision
to others in the organization. Keep telling people where you
want them to go. Keep telling them your vision of a New American Hospital. Keep telling them how important they are to the
process. Many New American Hospital executives have established an Executive Vision Council in order to provide a structure to accomplish this work. They say, "I can't do your job, but I
can tell you where we're going and how well we're getting there."
First we enunciate the dreams; then we set the targets.

Change Management Titles

How can we get our hospital managers to start thinking differently about their role? One positive sign has been the wide-scale
desertion of the dead term *administrator* in favor of *president* and
other corporate titles. That's a step in the right direction, but
how about pushing the creativity? One hospital president has
taken upon himself the title of Chief Servant — he's still the chief,
but his primary role is to serve. He says, "It created a very
interesting problem for my vice presidents. They couldn't figure
out how they could be called a vice president reporting to a
Chief Servant!" Or consider the new title given to supervisors at
Ford — team adviser. It puts the team first and then says that the
role of the boss is to advise the team.

One approach to retitling is to let managers create their
own titles. Keep the personnel people out of this — nothing is
going to change in terms of the salary! A title costs nothing, but
it is important and significant to the title holder. There's no
magic in a title; however, if it represents the new direction the
organization is taking, it can be a powerful symbol.

Openness to Criticism and Participation

In undertaking the conversion to the New American Hospital,
executives are empowering their managers to take action. In the

process, a number of programs near and dear to the executive heart will come under fire. These criticisms bring to the surface what everybody at the operating level knows—that these programs are inadequate, inaccurate, and nonproductive. The executive has to listen and not take these comments personally. It takes tremendous strength of ego to begin such a program, and even more to sustain it. As change moves forward, the executive role becomes one of being supportive of these new ventures, even if it is the executive's own pet ox that gets gored in the process. One of the real tests for the executive team during organization development is how much they can stand having nearly every decision and program they were ever part of criticized and torn apart.

The change process also calls for a lot of participation. Autocratic executives are going to be in for a much more difficult and unpleasant time than those who are more participative. One of the real keys to success is for the executive team to show an openness to criticism. They must also be supportive of changes that not all of their staff are going to be happy about.

Have Vice Presidents Work Their Areas

One of the new learnings at the vice presidential level is to cross the barriers that separate them from their own departments. Walt Disney instituted a practice where each August, executives were assigned to parking cars, taking tickets, serving hot dogs, even cleaning the toilets. He said, "If you don't see this business at the level the Customer sees the business, you don't understand the business." He wasn't interested in punishing his vice presidents, but in having them truly understand the problems the organization presents to its Customers. If you're an executive assigned to clean toilets and you can't lay your hands on the cleaner because the supply system isn't working, one of the things you are definitely going to do in September is fix that problem!

Similarly, hospital vice presidents do not understand the business. This comes about because of the normal separation that exists between executives and the actual work carried on in the departments. The problem is exacerbated since most hospital vice presidents did not come up through the ranks by internal promotion. It is the executive's job to bridge this gap. Requiring leaders to work in their departments for one month a year (or some other substantial, scheduled amount of time) gives impetus to the change effort and increases the leaders' stature. When people see leaders who are willing to do workaday jobs, it results in an immediate increase in respect. As the executive crosses the chasm of indifference, Associates begin to teach him the realities of the business. The universal experience of executives returning from these important sabbaticals is that they almost immediately change dozens of inadequate procedures!

By example, executives are teaching department heads that they, too, must cross the chasms of indifference, apathy, and ignorance. Associates who see leadership of that sort also know that this is a leader who "would never ask you to do anything he wouldn't himself." People feel closer to that kind of leadership. Being down in the trenches puts the leader into a situation where she is learning more about the business than could ever be learned in the office.

Too many hospitals are administered by remote-control executives, reading their *Wall Street Journal* with no understanding of work process. This leadership is phony; its decisions awful. American executives have a great deal to learn, much of it concerning the operations they're responsible for. Breaking down the barriers between leaders and led is an essential piece of executive work.

Get Executives Out of Operations

In the old hierarchy, hospital executives were little more than supermanagers. They routinely reviewed all departmental recommendations as well as siphoning off all the really enjoyable and interesting projects. As a result, department managers were crippled and trained not to take initiative.

To break this dependent role, and to force executives to do the work of top managing instead of vocational hobbying on departmental problems, specify that their role will not include involvement in department operations. While general oversight of departments remains, it should include only major policy changes, budget approvals, and resolution of major problems. The general rule should be that internal departmental and interdepartmental problems will be solved by the managers of those departments without executive interference.

Redefining the Management Mission

It's been said that *boss* is a four letter word—double S.O.B. spelled backward. The day of "superiors" and authoritarian leadership is over. It may still be widely practiced, but it is no longer viable. A new managerial role requires that department managers and supervisors work as the center of organizational renewal. With them, there is hope for revitalization; without them, there is no chance of a positive future for the organization.

Creative Destroyer, Hit Man of the Useless

Irwin Schumpeter, the American economist, used the phrase "creative destruction" to describe the state of desirable change. What do we want our managers to do? Do we want them to continue to placidly administer things as they are? Or do we want them to create something new and better? The answer is easy, but it is the sword side of creation that makes some executives nervous. If you want managers to create, they must be allowed to use their power to destroy. One hospital has officially given the names of Change Master and Creative Destroyer to all members of management!

Recently I asked a group of managers to identify fixable problems that their Customers have to suffer through, things that everybody knows need to be dealt with. In twenty minutes they identified forty items, some of which had been complaints for decades. When I asked why these problems had lingered so long, the lame answer was that they weren't anyone's direct responsibility. Isn't it obvious that we need a roving band of men and women who will take out the trash and kill off the problems that irritate Customers, eat budgets, and consume career lives?

Some very creative hospital presidents have even posted

"Wanted Dead or Alive" posters. Declare open season on the problem of your choice. Give cash rewards for meetings that are canceled and problems that are solved. Spread the concept to Associate levels. Put a bounty of one hundred dollars on any form that can be killed off or combined with another one, and watch the secretaries attack! One hospital even evaluates managers every ninety days on the number of "kills" and "zaps" they have achieved.

Throw Out Management Job Descriptions

Things are in transition. Don't try to keep management job descriptions accurate. Remember what Robert Townsend said about job descriptions in *Further Up the Organization*:

> Great for jobs where the turnover is high and the work is largely repetitive. Insane for jobs that pay $500 a week or more. Judgment jobs are constantly changing in nature and the good people should be allowed to use their jobs and see how good they are.
>
> At best, a job description freezes the job as the writer understood it at a particular instant in the past. At worst, they're prepared by personnel people who can't write and don't understand the jobs. Then they're not only expensive to prepare and regularly revise, but they're important morale-sappers.[2]

In the New American Hospital, the job description for everybody in management is (1) live the values and (2) achieve the seven KRAs.

Make Decisions at the Lowest Possible Level

Whose job is management? Not every task that involves a management principle should be done by a manager. No hospital could survive for long if every economic, productivity, or quality question was handled only by executives. In the New American

Hospital, dozens of new tasks will be given to managers and supervisors as they begin the process of download delegation. In turn, middle- and lower-level supervisors will have to download or offload the tasks they've previously been doing—that is, they must delegate much of their current job and, better yet, zap big chunks of needless work.

This requires a willingness to rethink who does what, who ought to, and why. It is absolutely unnecessary to have any requisition signed by more than two people, yet worker-years are spent in hospitals with redundant signature requirements. It is absolutely unnecessary to limit any manager to a spending authority of only a few hundred dollars, yet that is still routinely done in many hospitals. It is absolutely unnecessary for house-keeping supervisors to inspect every room. The job of inspecting a person's work belongs to the person who performed it, with only random verification necessary, yet mindless checking and rechecking still goes on.

I've tried this thought provoker on hospital management audiences:

> You have just received a new policy pronouncement signed by the president. It directs that from now on, any quality control issue or problem is to be solved only by hourly workers. No member of management can be involved in quality management. You have no choice but to abide by this directive. However, the president has asked you to be on a task force advising him how this crazy idea should be implemented to avoid possible disastrous consequences.

The reaction is always the same. Managers initially believe that it can't be done, but in twenty minutes of discussion they convert to precisely this radical position. Why? They realize that the action plan to implement this policy would require them to give Associates training support, checklists, clear standards of performance, and authority to take corrective action. And once that work has been done, it becomes painfully obvious that the board's crazy position is the only sane one.

Managers are not paid to do work. They are paid to get results. Far too many managers foolishly and compulsively take whatever work is dumped on their desk without thinking through the key question: Will this task contribute to the accomplishment of a KRA?

Download Delegation

There is no better way to force a realignment of job duties in the organization than by putting so much pressure on lower levels that they must, in turn, download decisions to others. As a vice president delegates not only work, but the authority and freedom to take action, and downloads decisions he or she formerly made to department heads, the department heads initially respond enthusiastically to this greater freedom. For a while they will attempt to maintain their job in its old format, in addition to taking on these newer executive duties. However, in time they come to the realization that they must eliminate some of these responsibilities by moving them down the organization or zapping them out of existence.

An important goal for executives and managers in the coming year is to make fewer decisions, not more; to handle fewer pieces of paper, not more; to go to fewer meetings, not more; to write fewer memos, not more. The watchword questions for all executives in this time period are: Why am I writing this memo, going to this meeting, making this decision? Why isn't somebody else doing it? Who could I train to do it? Who else should be doing it? The role of the executive now shifts to this downloading work, and to teaching department heads the principle of download delegation.

Create Constant Improvement of Service

Every job, every department, every manager, and every executive has one major goal: to improve service. Executives need to create a climate and an awareness that this improvement of service at all levels and in all things is the primary indicator of health in the organization. The executive war cry—Not good enough!—should be heard loudly and frequently through the organization. Even when work is accepted it ought to be accepted with the words: "It's good enough for now, but let's take another look at it in six months." Make the standard only temporarily acceptable; teach that there is no end point. Too many managers believe that they've got everything in good shape and running acceptably. That's the beginning of failure.

Drive Out Fear

This message is key in making continuous improvement possible. One of the primary roles of the New American Hospital executive is to deal with the paranoia, fear, anxiety, uncertainty, and doubt that abound in the old hospital. At first, managers and Associates will not trust the new direction and will lack confidence. Part of this emotional reaction is a by-product of thirty years of mismanaging people under the old control model. These people have been victimized, and it is going to take considerable effort before their fear dissipates. What this means is that executives must engage in hand holding, counseling, and encouraging others to take risks.

In one hospital, a department manager had courageously gone forth and done what needed to be done, only to have her peers immediately begin whispering that the sky was about to fall on her. The hospital president was furious. He simply could not believe that in an advanced stage of the organization's development, people could still be so filled with paralyzing fear. At the next department head meeting, the president had the department manager come forward. Turning to her he said, "Everyone is sure I'm going to give you the ax, but I'm not." Digging into his pocket, he took out two tickets to Bermuda, which he gave to her and her husband for a week's vacation. Then, turning to the astonished management group, he said, "Perhaps now you begin to get the message. Risk taking will not be punished here; it will be rewarded. Those of you who think or speak otherwise are not acting like members of this team. And, while this leader and her husband are enjoying Bermuda this weekend, I hope you enjoy staying here!"

Strong statements and symbolic actions are useful in breaking the logjam of fear. Don't underestimate how strong these forces are, or how paralyzing they are when people are trying to make organizations change. One of the key messages is that it's okay to make a mistake. Identify those who intimidate others and silence them. Identify the restraining factors and remove them.

Demand Management Transformation

Organizations have a pace and a tempo. In some organizations the tempo is a funeral dirge; in others it's Jumpin' Jack Flash! In every meeting and memo, let there be a continuing executive message on the need to transform the organization. Send a drumbeat through the jungle. Make people begin to understand that this is serious, that the transformation is going to occur, and that it's going to occur with them or without them. Don't equivocate about this or confuse people by pulling your punches.

Managers need to be aware of the real career risk in not making the crossover to the new philosophy and practice. While the basic culture should be supportive and encouraging, the message "buy in or bug out" needs to be sent, too. At one hospital, inside management's humor chant at meetings was "Change, Change, or Leave!" We want to drive out the fear that accompanies change, but there also ought to be fear of not changing. This simultaneous loose-tight message is akin to what I call Mom Management—she loved you, but she was the first to tell you to shape up!

Leadership Symbols and Behavior

What a leader does speaks more loudly than what she says. And the behavior that is most helpful in setting the leadership direction is symbolic. The effective leader asks: What can I do that would clearly let people know what I expect and stand for?

What Is Leadership?

Leadership is the ability to attract followers. If people are willing to follow you and your plan, you are a leader, even if you don't have a title or formal authority over them. If people are not willing to follow you, then you can have the biggest management title in the world and it will do you no good. Leadership is a question of what works with the followers. And that makes leadership style questions almost meaningless in terms of what a manager plans to do with the followers. The power is in the people, not in the manager.

What do people need in a leader? When asked to describe the "best leader I ever knew," followers describe two basic dimensions that must be present to some considerable degree in any manager who hopes to gain followership:

1. *Consideration.* The best leaders were described as caring, concerned, and two-way communicators. They supported people in the clinches, acted ethically, and showed respect to their followers. They expressed confidence and built follower self-esteem. They were often described as co-workers, cooperators, and collaborators, as being close, in contact, and able to establish rapport. Some leaders' manner was soft and warm; others practiced tough love. If the follower perceived that the leader was acting out of consideration, almost any style could be tolerated, gruff or gentle.
2. *Structure.* The best leaders set goals, objectives, and deadlines. They defined roles and removed ambiguity from people's work lives. These leaders set very high standards and expected people to meet them. They enforced these standards and disciplined people for mediocrity, not permitting them to be satisfied with less than their best. They were described as strong and decisive; they took positions and gave direction to the chaos around them. Whether the leader provided the structure directly or allowed followers to participate in setting their own structure, the end result was the same — direction.

Leaders should worry less about their stylistic approach and focus primarily on fulfilling followers' needs. Ask yourself if people in your organization need more consideration. Do they need more structure? Most leaders provide moderate consideration and moderate structure. As a result, their organizations are only moderately successful. What is called for is a substantial, intense investment in people along both dimensions. Excellent organizations have leaders high in consideration and structure, yet most hospital managements only score in the middle range on these dimensions.

Much of what has been termed situational leadership really has to do with what fits the audience. Young research scientists probably would not respond to too much overt control, but they would respond to a request for personally developed research objectives and standards. Soldiers on a battlefield in the midst of an artillery attack will not be interested in a participative approach to problem solving—they need direct and immediate orders. Find out what fits the situation and the needs of the people in the situation. Worry less about style, and more about communicating consideration and structure.

MBWA as the New Leadership Approach

"Managing by wandering about" was popularized by David Packard of Hewlett-Packard. It has also long been the operating approach of some of the most successful leaders and organizations. Wal-Mart Stores requires its executives to visit all stores each year to see directly what's going on and to respond to the needs they learn of firsthand. Bill Marriott does the same thing, as does Forrest Mars, Jr., of Mars, Inc. You can't manage an organization by sitting in an office. You've got to see what's going on and manage by using a hands-on approach. It is essential to realize that too many managers are out of touch with their Associates and Customers. They operate from reports and sit in meetings rather than confronting reality. MBWA has several key elements:

1.   MBWA is not aimless wandering; it is wandering with a purpose. Take one problem and ask everyone you see what

they advise should be done. Talk only with people who have been there a long time, or only with women, or gain the perspective of some other subgroup. Sometimes MBWA can take the form of a general bull session in the cafeteria, but it is never totally unplanned or mindless.

2. Set a certain percentage of time that will be spent in purposeful MBWA. A number of teams have set an MBWA performance expectation of 10 percent of the hours worked, 50 percent for executives. Experience shows that unless a time standard is set, leaders will stay in their offices, where their no-show behavior will remain part of the problem. Some will say that they haven't the time because of meetings and paperwork, to which effective leaders respond, "I haven't got the time for meetings and paperwork!" One of the best definitions of leadership is how you allocate your calendar.

3. Ask lots of tough questions; listen for the answers. Don't just wander through and say, "Hi!" That's MBWT, "managing by walking through." Use the time to get information, make notes, and start a dialogue.

4. Don't tell people how to do their job or try to answer questions on the spot. And don't undercut the chain of command. Whatever answers you provide should come after the visit when you've had a chance to think, and they should be transmitted through the chain of command.

5. On each visit, focus on a few key subjects, usually strategic objectives that are important to the business. In this informal exchange you can't deal with more than a few targets. Also, this type of focus teaches the organization what they should be concerned about—the word will get around that on this trip you were talking to everybody about higher quality, or training needs, or Customer service.

6. Realize that people will not be comfortable at first. They have to be given time to relax. Visit frequently, often enough so that people don't think twice about your presence. Always dress comfortably and informally to psychologically minimize the difference in status.

People incorrectly think MBWA is good because they see humanism in it. While there are good human values associated with such a practice, its primary good is to gather information directly and quickly. It keeps everybody honest since they know the boss is going to find out anyway!

How can you go directly to the troops? What forums and avenues can you use, and what messages do you want to give? In the midst of organizational change, people wonder where leaders stand and how committed they are. Tell them, and tell them to their face. Use formal meetings if you must, but rely more on discussions in the cafeteria. Show up at midnight with pizza for the night shift. Speak passionately and deeply; penetrate the blasé resistance of the tired soldiers who've heard it all before. If you want to be a leader, get out in front of the followers where they can see you. People don't follow a memo. They will only follow you.

Foster Open Communication

In open communication, people can know anything they want to know. There are no limits with the exception of personal and confidential matters. This means that the strategic plan and financial and competitive information are made available to everyone. Is this heresy?

The New American Hospital is a family. I don't know about your family, but there aren't any secrets in mine! I find that the minute you try to have one it sets off a lot of extra questions: "What's in that box? Is it for me?" People at work are a lot more paranoid. They assume that if you're not talking, you're hiding. Trust erodes, and there goes the ball game.

New American Hospitals communicate everything, and in a dynamic, effective way. Minutes of supervisory meetings and financial reports are posted for all to see. Large bulletin boards are used as communication centers in every department and in public areas. Management communicates useful, core information, instead of just low-level detail. This is supplemented by real give-and-take meetings, not one-way announcement sessions.

Letters to the newsletter editor don't only contain the safe questions with the milksop answers.

Every organization executive I ever talked with thinks that he or she makes a good effort at communication. Ask yourself some test questions: Could an Associate attend management meetings if she wanted to? Could a manager invite himself to a board meeting? Do managers leave work out on their desk for anyone to read, with notes asking for ideas on particular problems? If you believe that you have an open-door policy, take the doors off as they have at some hospitals. Stop talking about how much you believe in communication, and start changing the architecture!

Reduce Barriers Between the Leaders and the Led

Status differentials may be gratifying to the insecure, but they wreak havoc on a team. Do we really want those in management authority to have it so good that all others are peons by comparison? If you want to lead by example, you have to set an example. Maybe the time has come to stop the catered meals, the separate dining facilities, and the country club memberships. Some would rather have privilege than results.

Reduction of status differentials is not meant to take away rewards for achievement, but to reduce the barriers that separate the leaders from the led. This can take as simple a form as refusing to require people to call you "Mr." or "Ms." Would any leader who really wants open communication insist on a formal title that acts as a barrier? One way to view this minimization of status differential is to see that it doesn't lower executives as much as it raises up Associates.

Manage Like Sam Walton

One of the simplest conceptions of a business was the one put forward by Sam Walton, founder of Wal-Mart. He believed that a business is composed of three groups of people—Customers, Associates, and managers. The Customers have the money and are to be served. Their problem is that they sometimes have difficulty getting what they want (it's out of stock; they have to wait too long for it). Associates are on the payroll to give Customers what they want. They experience another set of problems as they try to serve the Customers' needs (they have too much paperwork; the stock cart is broken). The problems experienced by Customers and Associates are the reason management is needed.

What is management supposed to do? Three things. First, *listen.* Listen to Customers and Associates, to their problems and needs. At Wal-Mart this requires 80 percent of an executive's time. MBWA requires time, and the purpose is not to be seen as the leader sitting in an office and reading reports that never capture the truth of what's happening, but to spend time where the action is. The second requirement is to *believe.* Rather than discounting what the Customer says, or thinking that the Associate is overstating things in order to gain personal advantage, why not just believe what is being said? Even taking into account distortions in communication most people are telling you the truth most of the time. The third function of management is to *do.* Do what you've been told is needed by the Customer. Do what the Associate says would help to get things done.

An example of the new leadership was provided to me by a young assistant vice president. It was the first year of her new job. She asked what I thought of the idea of spending time working in each of her departments. Since she obviously knew what was needed, I asked what concerned her about doing it. "Well, none of the other vice presidents do that here, and I don't want to look foolish, either to them or to my departments." As we talked through her concerns, she finally decided to take the risk and go ahead.

Her first task was to work in the kitchen, where she was assigned to the senior baker. She was given the job of filling breakfast rolls with custard. It took her the better part of a week to master this skill. All around her, Associates were watching and talking. They joked with her about her many failures with the custard press. They admired her grit and sense of humor, and they began to accept her desire to understand.

The story spread through the hospital grapevine. It even

made the front page of the community newspaper. Think of it—
an executive who wasn't afraid to get her hands dirty, and who
thought that listening to "hourlies" was an important thing to do!
Associates from other departments began to seek her out. So,
too, did Associates who reported to other executives. She was
fast becoming the "people's executive." Her power in the informal world increased almost exponentially. People told her about
their situation and her understanding of the inner workings of
the organization increased, so that her recommendations became more sensible and powerful.

The power of any leader always and ultimately comes
from the followers. This isn't just a democratic ideal; it is management reality.

Build Muscle on the Management Team

A major cause of poor organizational functioning is the inade-
quacy of present procedures to select supervisors, an absence of
management development and grooming, poor performance of
the management job itself, and the accumulation of deadwood
and defenders of managerial fiefdoms. How should this problem be corrected where it exists, and how can good managers be
supercharged?

The leadership of the New American Hospital needs to
reflect the organization's new realities and operating environment. New American Hospital leaders will both change the
organizational environment and be changed by it. The only
effective leadership style is the one that is appropriate to the
situation, and the situation now requires a more human and
participative approach to leading people toward functioning
more effectively.

The situation has changed, and it is important not to try
to play the new management game by the old rules. Executives
who fail to make this transition will have profound difficulties
politically as they elicit poor economic and service performance
from their staff. Indeed, this may be one of those situations
where we are led by events more than we lead them.

The Old Model

When the concept of the physician as administrative leader of the hospital began to break down in the 1930s, no trained managerial cadre existed to pick up the reins. Master of hospital administration (M.H.A.) programs began to fill the gap. However, unlike other industries in late twentieth-century America, the M.H.A.-trained group maintained its insularity from lower management levels. It is rare in hospitals for a department head to be able to move into a top-level position and the normal pattern used by successful organizations of moving people up from the ranks is missing.

The maintenance of this truncated management ladder has a negative impact that threatens the ability of a hospital to become a New American Hospital. First, middle managers are not ready to assume higher responsibility. Years of career neglect and absence of management development work produce managers who do not have advanced understanding of the larger management processes that must now be directed anew. Second, there is a middle-management malaise, a sense of low expectations and low morale. As one hospital president described it, "Managers for years were trained to be passive dependent, not aggressively interdependent or independent."

As if these problems were not enough, executive ranks within the current hospital model are all too often "free-floating apexes." They have formal titular authority, but they are remote from understanding the technical workings of the departments they supervise, and they lack the history and feel of the managerial underground. Such executives are unable to control except by fiat and tight review.

Lest the reader think otherwise, let me state my observation of the brightness of young hospital executives. It's not their fault that the situation they have inherited is as it is. But it is their generation that will have to reconsider and redesign the way in which management talent is identified, developed, and promoted.

Select or Correct

Improve the Selection Processes. Do you have the right people in the right jobs, and what do you do if you don't? In the past most supervisors and department heads were selected based on either greater seniority or technical expertise. The research indicates that these variables are not related to effective managerial performance. Sometimes an average nurse is by temperament and aptitude the best candidate for a supervisory position. It is important to immediately choke off the fuzzy thinking that allows the promotion of the halfhearted and half-witted. In the New American Hospital, leadership, not administration, is the primary arena for action. The hospital whose management team is able to mobilize and multiply the brain-power and energies of its human resources is the hospital that wins. Therefore, leadership capability will be the key criterion by which hospital managers will be selected in the future.

In the past it was thought that just throwing people into the swimming pool would work as an approach to promoting managers; they would sink or swim. Unfortunately, what a lot of hospitals got was nonsinkers, not championship swimmers. The New American Hospital is successful to a large measure because its defensive screens protect it from those who are unqualified to manage. Such aggressive selection processes also create an awareness that management positions aren't inherited; they come from being good at the job. This generates in turn a pride of position that too often is lacking in losing organizations.

In a number of hospitals, management selection now follows a much more systematic process, including use of such tools as posting all management jobs, multiple interviews with multiple interviewers (including some outside of the division and chain of command to represent team viewpoints), ratings from both peers and subordinates, and presupervisory train-ing. If this sounds like work, it is. But it is a lot less work than trying to clean up the mess made by bad supervisors.

Select Leaders, Not Managers. Organizational change is primarily a human leadership challenge. We no longer need more administrators. The industry has been administered into a coma. Today's task is to find men and women who are truly qualified to be leaders of people engaged in a major effort to change and improve their organizations.

An excellent example of this occurred at one hospital where the president called me asking for a formal psychological assessment to confirm his selection of a new vice president of finance. I asked him whether he was going outside to find someone for the position. The president said, "No, I'm promoting from within." I said, "Oh, a member of the accounting staff, no doubt." He replied, "No, he's not a member of the accounting staff, has never taken a course in accounting, does not have a degree in accounting, finance, or any related discipline, and is currently our director of physical therapy." I said, "Well, that's certainly a nontraditional approach — teach me." He answered, "What's wrong in that department is that people do not trust administration. They've been intimidated and are afraid to make decisions on their own. I have some good accountants, but frankly, accountants are a dime a dozen. I don't need another accountant, I have plenty of people down there who can give me the technical answers. What I need is a leader."

When he was tested, this fellow scored as high in leadership capability as any candidate I've seen. His first decision in the job was to immediately move his office from the remote executive carpetland down to an open area in the middle of the accounting unit so that he could be with the people. In less than six months the staff had fully turned around in their attitudes and morale. The selection simply could not have been better. Coming from a nontraditional background, he had no preconceived notions of what would or would not work. This also meant that he was open to receiving the ideas of his subordinates. Because of his lack of financial training, he had to take upon himself the role of learning most of the technical aspects of the job from his direct reports, all of whom were highly qualified technically. Only those leaders whose minds are open, and who believe that people are more important than the work that they do, can effectively lead organizational change.

Promote from Within: Just Say No to Inexperience. To lead a hospital through the trauma of the next decade, members of the executive team must be experienced risk takers. Young M.H.A.'s fresh out of school should no longer be hired as vice presidential candidates. The industry simply can no longer afford to give them a job as the number-two or number-three person in the hierarchy while they go through basic training. Hospitals must follow the usual career path used by all successful organizations, in which experienced department heads are promoted internally. Those who have risk-taking ability, entrepreneurial experience, and the necessary street smarts will succeed in the new environment. Those who entered health care administration thinking that it was a relatively no-risk job, and who are fearful of command decision-making power, should not be considered for a position regardless of the quality of their academic résumé.

When the organization cannot find adequate management talent in-house (this problem should be considered a short-term situation, not one that will be allowed to persist), hiring experienced risk takers from the outside makes the most sense. This process is already well under way in the industry, with a considerable number of experienced executives and management personnel being brought in from other industries and backgrounds. I would prefer to see the organization eventually become able to breed its own management talent, but for now, bringing people in who do not suffer from industry "groupthink" may be the best approach. Don't add to your problems by hiring too variant a group of top- and middle-management people. A high variation in the top levels makes subsequent organization development work extremely difficult. Find the new blood needed, and get the transfusion going!

Use Management Development as a Change Arena

Owners rarely draft a finished, fully developed player in the NBA or NFL, and it's unlikely that even good selection will net a fully developed manager. Rookies need to go to preseason training, and managers, too, need to learn their craft. Yet studies of management development as a change strategy show that very little behavioral change results from such programs. This low level of impact on change (about 5 to 7 percent) occurs because the organization's culture punishes new ideas. As a consequence, I advise organizations to stop doing supervisory training and management development until they are willing and able to make organizational change. Unless you are willing to start doing things differently in the hospital, don't talk about doing things differently in the classroom. The assumption that giving new ideas to managers will cause them to manage differently has been disproved, so why spend money and frustrate managers?

On the other hand, imagine what happens in an organization where top leadership commits to the idea of organizational renewal and openly encourages managers to criticize and improve the system. A tremendous morale uplift comes from eliminating long-standing problems, and an exciting team spirit results from joining together in a common cause. As new practices and norms are created by the group, a tougher and more dedicated team results.

Management development should be used as the channel to drive organization development. It's a bit of a gamble to trust managers this much — what if they start throwing those grenades at the policy *you* wrote! In fact, this process never backfires, because managers want to win and they want to help their organization win. As one hospital president told me, "It's never a gamble to bet on the basic goodness of people and their desire to win. The real gamble would be to not give them a voice." (See Chapter Eleven, for a full discussion of how this is done.)

Identify and Remove Manager Blockages

During the management development sessions, a long list of barriers and blockages are identified that interfere with the manager's job. These are usually real problems, not just excuses. As they come to light, executives should take immediate action to get rid of them. Managers are being asked to take new risks and believe in the new vision — they need proof that executives are doing more than talking. Executives who help remove blockages are expressing their commitment forcefully, and that begins the process of belief on the part of their managers.

When managers are asked to list and prioritize their barriers, they may pick items that don't seem all that important. Maybe it's spending authority, or the ability to replace a budgeted position without getting a second approval. Whatever the item is, fix it. In some cases the issue may be something big, like disciplining the hospital's most important physician for staff abuse. This is the executive test. Will she or won't she respond? If she doesn't cross that line, the program is dead. The Praetorian Guard were loyal to Caesar because he backed their play.

Build the Team by Confronting Resistance

A whole host of barriers exist in most management teams—old enmities, positions, impressions, or attitudes. These can best be attacked tangentially. When managers see that the vast majority of their peers are too busy having a good time, it's a lot harder for them to find someone to complain with. By letting the group norm move away from the noncooperative complainer, that person is isolated. This creates a pressure that will either suppress this behavior or make it stand out starkly as not fitting in.

If the team-building effects of socialization and problem solving are insufficient to draw all factions into the team, tougher approaches may be necessary. I counsel executives to wait for the new group norms to form, and then to confront the troublemakers, either individually or by making reference to the faction in a larger meeting. Some growth comes on its own, and some comes from a clear statement by the executive as to what is expected. It may be necessary to tell troublemakers to stop if they aren't bright enough to understand what's happening around them. Low-structure executives shrink from this task; high-structure leaders do not.

Usually dissatisfaction with poor performers originates within a group when the complaint is raised that not all managers are moving in the new direction. This complaint can be constructively handled by asking a subgroup to create a list of the managerial behaviors that are now considered unacceptable to the team. When a list of twenty items goes up on the screen, the managers affected can be seen to squirm. This is the voice of the group sending a warning to the few. I will often ask the question, "Today the group is speaking about what it doesn't want to see around here anymore. What do you think will happen if a manager is still doing these things in a year?" Invariably, the group response is, "They won't be here." The organization's mission is too important to sacrifice to the inability of the few to adapt. The day is past when a hospital dedicated to winning the playoffs will tolerate nonteam behaviors.

Remove Uncommitted Problem Managers

Managers who are not able to make the trip shouldn't start the journey. If some managers have not grown with their peers, if at the end of management training they have not been able to adapt to the new culture, then it's time to remove them. The executives who provided the growth opportunity have now done all they can to reprogram these people. Now is the time to recognize that the developmental approach did not work for them. My experience is that there are never more than a few of these people, but there always are some. Ask yourself this question: With the kind of organization we've been building, would I hire this person for a management job today? If the answer is no, you know what has to be done.

As it becomes clear that people do not have the inclination, talent, or willingness to learn, they should be removed. Do this as soon as possible, so as not to hamper the organizational change processes. Perhaps they'd be good as a technician in their original area of training. Perhaps it's time for them to leave the organization altogether. Our experience suggests that this group will consist of between 5 and 10 percent of the managers. Remember, you can't have a winning team with losing coaches. With problem managers removed, reward loyal supporters with additional responsibilities. Begin regrouping departments by giving them to those who have been strong in the battle.

Notes

1. A. Toffler, *Power Shift* (New York: Bantam Books, 1990), p. 28.
2. R. Townsend, *Further Up the Organization* (New York: Harper-Collins, 1970), p. 115.

9

Managing
Wide-Scale Change
and Reconstruction

Action. This day.
— Winston Churchill's
standard memo opening

Leading an organization through renewal requires careful thought about the sheer magnitude of change that will be attempted. How do leaders at all levels encourage a climate and culture for change? Substantial planning for the change will be required rather than shooting from the hip. Leaders can manage the identified elements of a formula for change. Once the change process is under way, driving change with value-centered management will be necessary to keep things on-track and moving forward. Finally, all of this needs to be reduced to an action plan for change that will take place in *three waves*: *preparation*, *implementation*, and *acceleration*.

The Magnitude of Organizational Change

Organizational changes of the dimension envisioned in the New American Hospital mean nothing less than a complete overhaul of everything that is done to manage the organization. This overhaul requires the overthrow of most policies and practices and an almost complete reversal of existing beliefs and attitudes about how work should be done, Customers served, and Associates utilized.

As if that were not enough, these changes will be installed in a climate of confusion and chaos, with the potential of wide--

185

scale resistance. But the New American Hospital knows that the lodestar of change, its guiding beacon, must be the voice of the Customer, a voice echoed in the commonsense intelligence of Associates struggling to serve under the rigid rules that the old hospital substitutes for getting results.

Management Change Myopia

Few managements have come to grips with the nature of the change problem facing American hospitals. They have not:

- Understood that they are dealing with a massive change need, one that will not respond to a few program add-ons
- Comprehended that the nature of change itself has become revolutionary instead of evolutionary
- Seen that the major issue is not cost or volume, but the improvement of quality
- Realized the size of the target of opportunity—if they win the issue and make the change, they will prevail over competitors
- Understood that the pace of change in the hospital must rapidly accelerate despite the frenzy of change already going on, or realized that while old hospitals are moving, they're moving too slowly
- Recognized that people and systems, not capital and technology, are the key to success

The management of change is the defining critical skill for managers in an era of explosive change. In earlier days, there was time to react. Today, managers must deal with greater amounts of change in a shorter time. Badly managed change concerning a new policy, project, or procedure can have disastrous effects on organizational functioning and the manager's reputation. The key test of effective managers is whether they can gain acceptance for change and smoothly weave it into the organizational fabric.

Organizational Approaches to Change

The failure to recognize the fundamental shift in the nature of change can be seen in how old hospitals manage compared to the New American Hospital:

Old Hospital	*New American Hospital*
Approach to change:	*Approach to change:*
Hire consultant, diagnose and study	Ask the people, prescribe and fix
Have a bias for caution, consensus	Have a bias for action
Change the organizational design	Ignore the organizational structure
Revise the organizational chart	Publish all-inclusive phone books
Impose productivity, dollar limits	Develop people, resource control
Develop MIS for executive control	Establish information loops to managers and Associates
Be defensive, avoid failure	Take the offensive, seek success
Change the organization, get people to fit	Change people, fit the structure to them
Tap management's few brains	Tap Associates' many brains
Believe in past monoliths	Distrust or reject past dogmas

Change Assumptions and Practices

A different set of assumptions exists about the nature of change between old and new hospitals:

Old Hospital	*New American Hospital*
Change is seen as:	*Change is seen as:*
Linear, predictable	Nonlinear, multibranching
Evolutionary, continuous	Revolutionary, discontinuous

Volume difficult but acceptable	Volume out of control
Mechanical	Biological
Having to do with knowledge, being in control	Having to do with ignorance
Stable state, rigidity	Unstable state, thriving on chaos
Resisted, status quo defended	Welcomed, best defense is offense
Project by project	Emphasis on systems
Imitative — monkey see, monkey do	Original, home-grown, creative
Energy level low, drained	High energy output, fatigued

Old Hospital	*New American Hospital*
Change practices are:	*Change practices are:*
Program of the Month	Radical shift in culture
Few elitist brains, committees	Everyone in Do It Groups
Total Quality Management	Total Management, all KRAs
Lip service to vendor-purchased values	Articulated and enforced internal values
Herky-jerky patchwork	Comprehensive, systematic plan
Strategic planning	Strategic Customer response
Guest relations	Customer "Wow" service
Reactive, slow	Proactive, time-based
Wait for certainty	Make improvements today
Nice, neat, broke	Confusing, happy, profitable

Encouraging a Change Culture

The New American Hospital nourishes a climate of continuous change. Members say, "Let's try anything we can think of that has a reasonable chance." This means allowing people to break rules and do end runs around policy as they experiment. Leaders want some chaotic change and lots of new ideas. They're even willing to tolerate experiments others might think of as wacky, but at the same time they must maintain some control of the process — they can't let people get away with murder. And so, a dynamic tension is created. Every work situation is like a battle-field. The commanders who forget the book and do what the situation requires, who show creativity under pressure, are the ones who win the wars. At the same time, the commanders who only shoot from the hip and who are not disciplined in the art of war end in disaster. A balance is called for, one executed with boldness.

Nourish Creative Chaos in the Change Climate

Empower change champions. What label should be given to people in your organization who take risks for the sake of their ideas? One hospital refers to them as Crusader Rabbits. Another gives the Jack and Joan of Arc award. The nontraditional, nonex-isting idea must be given a place of honor within the organiza-tion. Create experiments everywhere. Give the assignment to any person or group eager to try a different idea. Bet on moti-vation, not job title or departmental appropriateness. The im-possible dream is often doable by the person of vision. Some efforts may fail, but enough successes will result to more than pay for the failures. It's better to have messy creativity that doesn't stay between the lines than orderly boredom.

Leaders need to ask the central question: Is our climate conducive to people wanting to make change? As change begins to roll out, various groups start their resistance. While mouthing support for the overall renewal, they take issue with the means, find a particular unsuccessful idea to publicize, and suggest that the organization "go slow." At this crucial juncture when the new change climate is not firmly entrenched, executives must con-tinue to voice dissatisfaction with the status quo and create a climate in which change is nurtured. One group will be very concerned with the sometimes chaotic nature of change; they are the neatness bugs who prize order more than results. Do not be thrown off by ideas that didn't work or political factions that may organize against it. Continue to push for change. Let it be known that those who push with you are going to be favored in the management hierarchy. Do not be naive in thinking that all you have to do is announce the renewal program and somehow it will magically happen. The hard work of driving the change into the culture now begins.

Too Little Isn't Enough

Don't underestimate the need to create a new management culture. More and more hospitals have now changed to the Associate label or adopted values statements. However, some-times a few surface pieces of the New American Hospital model are adopted without establishing the more substantial cultural elements, systems, and change mechanisms that make it all work. The temptation is to think that these few ideas are the solution, and that they're all that's necessary to make things change. Nothing could be further from the truth. This is lightweight thinking and dilettante behavior. How can organizations be shown that they must truly change, not simply add window dressing?

What must occur is the creation of a new management culture from the standpoint of how people respond and behave within it. For example, the values statement is simply a centering device that clarifies key expectations and authorities. Manage-ment must follow up with rewards and enforce sanctions against violators. Managers who assign new labels and make pro-nouncements about values but don't do the hard work that completes these ideas are playing at change management. They are not change masters; they are change amateurs.

Innovation Is Driven by Dissatisfaction

Only when there is dissatisfaction over the way things are will people begin to look for ways to make things better. Some sources of dissatisfaction are complaints from physicians, board members' anger over bad financial pictures, executive management's own position that things must change, opinion survey scores showing employees' low opinions of the work situation, and Customers who want to sue. The savvy management is the one that taps these sources to motivate the change process. It is important to highlight as many failings as possible. Point out what rival hospitals are doing that is clearly better than yours. Don't allow the organization to become satisfied and smugly content with what it is doing.

I remember consulting with an organization that had made a number of changes, resulting in above-average Customer ratings, but then had fallen into the complacency trap, stopping far short of what they might have been able to attain. Therefore, build in a continuing set of sources of dissatisfaction that never let people feel they have it made. As you roll out innovation and success, also roll out the message that there's still a lot of work to do.

Planning for Change

In getting started with planning change, whether it's as large-scale as an organizational renewal or as small as a departmental project, it's useful to think through the way that change will work in your particular situation. The following questions will help structure your thinking about change in your hospital.

Organizational History

Identify any significant history that will affect the change you are planning. What has happened in, around, or about the change arena that you will be operating in? What occurred in the past that will have a present impact? (Past events might include changes in management direction, competition, regulations, economics, morale, reporting relationships, new products, or consultant reports.)

To help your thinking, write down any significant recent or historical factor or event that should be considered. Ask what impact or influence it will have on the change you're planning to make.

Force-Field Analysis

Change always occurs in a force field. Certain forces push for the change, while other forces restrain it. First identify what these forces are, then devise a plan for dealing with them.

Driving forces are those that favor your change; they may include such things as the corporate culture; potential for profit; benefits and rewards; key sponsors; and powerful people; or the change may simply be popular. Identify and list all the driving forces operating in your situation. Are there other force factors that could be added to this list? Then, identify how each of them can be strengthened or their potential increased?

Restraining forces are those that resist the change. They may include such items as cost; lack of time; human insecurities; regulations, policies, and precedent; opposition or relationships of key players; or simple inertia. Now identify all the restraining forces. Can any of these forces be removed from the list or neutralized? How can the influence of those that remain be weakened or moderated? List the restraining forces, and then identify how each of them could be weakened or dealt with.

Test the Change Initiative for Fit

Look before you leap. Think through whether it's possible to make the change you're contemplating. There are three tests for fit, and a failure on any one could represent a failure for your planned change.

> *Test 1:* Is there a reasonable fit between the magnitude of the change being contemplated and your power in the organization? If not, is the change too big to be attempted? Can it be scaled down to a smaller change initiative?
>
> *Test 2:* Is there a reasonable fit between the model, vision, or goal of what is to be done, and the organizational

realities and imperatives that form the context of the change environment? (What is it possible to do, here, in terms of the change itself?) If not, can the model be changed?

Test 3: Is there a reasonable fit between internal change readiness on the part of key individuals and groups (their attitudes, skills, and dissatisfaction energy) and the change method you intend to use—either a *participative* approach (working on people's attitudes first, then installing the change) or a *directive* approach (making the change first, then working on people's attitudes)?

Managing the Change Formula

Studies of both successful and unsuccessful change initiatives show there are a number of factors that must be simultaneously managed. Will your proposed change measure up to the following formula?[1] Can you manage these different change elements? If not, serious trouble or failure could result. The formula is

$$C = D \times M \times P > \text{Costs}$$

where C = change, D = dissatisfaction/desire, M = model, and P = process. Change will occur only when each of the factors D, M, and P are present in sufficient degree. If any of these factors are absent or insufficient, change will not occur. In addition, the interaction of D, M, and P must be positive enough for the benefits of change to be greater than its costs. Costs are time, effort, and money, but more importantly, personal costs in terms of loss of confidence, competence, and relationships. Personal costs are always paid by those affected by the change.

Change most often occurs under conditions of dissatisfaction, not positive desire. D is the pressure to change, caused either by internal factors such as management or labor unrest or by external forces such as competition or governmental regulations. D is the energy needed for change to occur and is usually the result of a crisis, or of relevant, accurate, and politically supported data. A key role for the manager is to increase D in order to energize the organization for change. The change master asks, "How can I get people to be unhappy enough with the status quo that they'll want to change it?"

M is the vision of the new way of doing things, the new way of thinking, feeling, and behaving. Creating D without M leads to blame and accusations—people don't know what to do. Most managers provide M, an adequate picture or plan, but fall down in providing P.

P is the way in which individuals or groups affected by the change have a chance to work through their resistance and reach a point of buy-in. To process change requires communication, participation, and time. The usual mistakes are top-down or bottom-up processing in which higher or lower levels of the organization try to influence each other. The best approach, where time allows, is a cyclical P, where different levels lay out M and seek the reactions of others who are affected. Involvement almost invariably leads to buy-in. The old hospital either gave edicts (top-down) or asked for input it never used (bottom-up). The New American Hospital goes for cyclical processing at the lowest possible levels (DIGs), and uses top-down for change and values enforcement.

Dissatisfaction/Desire Must Be Generated

A few questions allow you to test whether you have provided adequately for all of the necessary factors involved in the change. Decide which factors need more work. First, besides yourself, who will provide the energy for change? Who is dissatisfied with the present situation or desires a better way? How can other personal energy sources be brought into play to increase D? What or who is going to drive the change through? A common failing is underestimating the amount of physical, emotional, and intellectual energy that change requires. Do you and others have the necessary staying power?

Second, ask how D can be communicated or spread in the system. In what creative ways can it be increased? What information or example would help spread D and win change adherents? What risks exist in increasing D?

Creating an Adequate Model

Ask: What is the M? What specific model, plan, or picture has been drawn up that specifies what the end result will be and how we get there step by step? How can this be clarified, simplified, and visualized? What needs to be done to improve the model?

Also ask whether implementation of the model can be staged or broken down into component parts to make communication or implementation easier. Can a pilot of the model be installed and tested rather than having to just jump into things? Who would champion and defend the pilot test from those who are against it?

Obtaining Buy-In from Stakeholders

P (processing) is the term that describes how people reach a point of buy-in. Can others be made stakeholders in the change? What part of the change can be made relevant to their interests? Can elements be negotiated—not compromised—to increase leverage on others to support the change?

What rewards and recognitions can be provided to induce or support compliance? How can rewards be reduced for other competing views? What's in it for those affected? Is an analysis of the stakeholders' position a good idea to determine what forces are affecting them? What glory can be shared?

Ask whether those who are affected will have a hand in shaping the model. Can they design it, test it, train in it before full implementation? Does their standing in the organization, skill level, or leadership affect this question?

Can the change be made fun, enjoyable, and positive? What subgoals or early results can be celebrated? How can the satisfaction of achievement be made available and real? Celebration throughout the change is essential—how will it be sustained?

Exhibit 9.1 provides an instrument with which you can assess whether your efforts at change will pay off.

Exhibit 9.1. The Benefit-Cost Ratio.

Change will usually occur only if the benefits of $D \times M \times P$ are greater than the costs. First, identify the benefits and costs of the change you're contemplating. Benefits might be related to economics, operating efficiency, personal or professional advancement, or competitive advantage. Costs might include such things as expense, time and effort, organizational paralysis, threat to personal status, job security, or competence. Next, assign a weighting of 1–10 points for each element (1 = low, 10 = high), and total the points to see if benefits exceed costs by a substantial margin.

Benefits	Points	Costs	Points
_____	_____	_____	_____
_____	_____	_____	_____
_____	_____	_____	_____
_____	_____	_____	_____
_____	_____	_____	_____
Total	_____	*Total*	_____

Dealing with Resistance

Resistance to change is normal and expected. While planning for processing will greatly reduce resistance, it's wise to plan on some problems arising. People resist change for predictable reasons. Some of those reasons are nonproductive and energy-sapping; some are good and sound. All of them must be managed to ensure implementation of the change initiative. Which of the following resistance factors will be a part of your change situation?

1. *Lack of understanding or poor communication*
    - Fear of the unknown
    - Not understanding the change or seeing the need for it

- Not liking the way in which the change was introduced
- Not being communicated with about the change or getting the news second-hand
- Inability to prepare; not knowing how to perform
2. *Losses or costs of change*
   - Perceived loss of job or relationships
   - Comfort in the present way of doing things
   - Feeling that the change will not be beneficial
   - Seeing too great a cost in terms of personal life, competence, confidence, or relationships
   - Fear of not fitting into the group norms or fear that acceptance of the change will lead to social isolation from one's peers
   - Thinking that tossing out the present system is a rejection of the self-investment and creativity put into the current method
3. *No participation or control*
   - Not being asked about the change—a feeling of being a cog in the machine
   - Giving minimal compliance or conformity; using passive resistance as a way to mask true feelings
4. *Attitudinal problems or emotional reactions*
   - Negative mind-set about the job or organization to begin with; expressing it by resisting
   - Change seen as personal criticism, a perceived slap at one's competence
   - Dislike of the person introducing the change; bad relationship history
   - Personal immaturity, or possession of a "bad attitude"
   - Defense reactions (rationalizing, delaying, projecting blame) to protect comfort in the status quo
   - Emotional coloring due to fear, anger, prejudice, frustration, hostility, insecurity, and resentment
5. *Legitimate work concerns*
   - Bad timing, too much on one's plate already; too much work to do
   - Insufficient resources or other causes of a perceived certainty of failure

- Change seen as incorrect or unethical, a violation of values
- Being told to change with no direction about what to do
- Change seen as overly complex or ambiguous, or with an inadequate implementation plan

If you feel that the above resistance factors should be prepared for in advance, create a three-column matrix. First, list the persons or groups you think will be resistant. Then list the factors that you think will cause this resistance. Finally, identify what approaches you will take to this resistance.

Driving Organizational Change with Values

Organizational change requires a tremendous amount of driving force and energy. Active resistance and the inertia of the status quo are enormous blocks to change. This is even more true when organizational renewal is undertaken because it seeks to make wide-scale change in a short period of time. Discover what forces can be marshaled to drive organizational change, because no change will happen without a tremendous amount of change energy to push it. By thinking intelligently about how to put change energy to work, we avoid burnout as change agents and win supporters in the process.

The Roman Empire was not built by the Caesars, but by the centurions. There was no time to write Rome a memo; decisions had to be made on the battlefield, and they had to be made immediately. How did Rome control its legions in the field? First, centurions took a personal oath to Caesar and the Empire. Second, they were trained in the skills of both warfare and civil administration. And third, they were commissioned to make decisions on the spot, and a sword was put into their hands!

A new generation of American hospital executives is returning to this ancient concept of decentralized, lower-level decision making. To do so, hospital managers sign a statement of commitment to the organization's values. They are trained to do the management job well, and their performance is evaluated to make sure that they understood the message. And then the payoff, the sword of managerial accountability, is put into their hands. How would you like to have such a team fighting for your interests?

Values-centered management, in its simplest conceptual form, means that control is effected by identifying the core values and areas of performance need. QSCV (Quality, Service, Cleanliness, and Value) is McDonald's approach to value-centered managing. This program is stressed to new employees in orientation and then tied to performance evaluation, pay increases, and promotions. Employees soon learn that QSCV is absolutely essential to getting ahead within the organization.

Using the Values Statement to Effect Change

Values-centeredness is important since the renewal program introduces a large amount of change into the organization. Managers and Associates alike need a values statement as a source of constancy of purpose in the midst of swirling and accelerating change. The values statement is not a slogan or gimmick, but a management tool to control decision making. Created by managers and approved by the chief executive, this action-oriented guide tells everyone what behaviors and decisions are acceptable — and which decisions represent violations of core values. In this way, the organization controls decision making while at the same time empowering employees to take action without waiting for approval. Most organizations link the values statement to merit pay, performance evaluations, and promotion review.

The values statement becomes a *driver* of change as staff use it to measure everything that they and others are doing. It acts as a *control* on staff whereby they can check on what they're doing. It *frees* up staff by letting them take action to make change. It *motivates* people in their pursuit of life's best values — a sacred quest. And it gives people a *stabilizer* to hang onto in the midst of change.

How to Create a Values Statement

How does one go about establishing a values-centered management approach while creating the climate necessary to sustain
it? It is always best to work with the existing culture and values
within the organization, rather than trying to implant them
artificially. The worst counterfeit is the use of vendor values, in
which a guest relations program bought from an outside vendor
provides a values statement that has nothing to do with the
history of the organization. Like foreign tissue, the host may
soon reject it.

How is a values statement created? In some organizations,
top management has taken the responsibility for enunciating
the values statement. In other cases it has been handled by a
group of combined top and middle managers in a seminar
setting. Still other organizations have gone to the unnecessary
length of hiring values consultants and surveying various con-
stituency groups. My experience is that the values are readily at
hand and can be quickly created by the organization. Some of
the statements hospitals have created include:

- QUEST: Quality, Unity, Empathy, Service, Tradition
- SPIRIT: Serve, Performance, Integrity, Respect, Innovation,
  Team
- ESPRIT: Excellence, Service, People, Responsibility, Innova-
  tion, Team
- SERVE: Service, Enthusiasm, Respect, Value, Excellence
- PRIDE: People serving people, Respect for all, Improving
  constantly, Do it now, Excellence
- CARE: *Customer:* Always First; *Actions* Speak Louder Than
  Words; *Respect* = the Golden Rule; *Excellence* Is Our Standard

Notice how independent teams tend to identify similar
values. In most cases managers are able to construct an acronym
in thirty minutes or less. In a few cases the group process doesn't
click, and more work is required. That it works so successfully
most of the time is because the organization's values are already
present. The acronym is only an articulation process.

Testing the Statement

Since the objective is to create a working tool, any values statement needs to pass several tests:

- Is it understandable? Are the words simple and clear?
- Are the words guides to daily decision making? *Serve* and *respect* are words that pass this test. Words like *attitude, enthusiasm,* or *hope* are less helpful in telling people what to do.
- Do the words apply to all jobs? Do they cover the work done by both executives and salad makers?
- Is the values statement memorizable? Three to five words are; eight are too many. If it can't be memorized, it won't be used.
- Does the statement have punch? Are the words motivating?
- Does it include *serve* (implies focus on the Customer), *respect* (relations with Associates), and *excellence* (the level at which work is to be done), or their synonyms? These concepts were most frequently found in the values statements of the excellent companies and are most central to effective organizational functioning.

It's a good idea to test the values statement with several reference groups before publication. Perhaps the most important group is the Associates. If they understand the statement's meaning and how it would apply to their job, you've got something! Some organizations have also tested their statement in Customer or physician focus groups to see if they can understand it. Keep in mind, however, that this is a tool for internal management, not for other purposes. It does not replace the organization's mission statement or statements of belief by religious sponsors, and is not a marketing slogan.

Implementing the Values Statement

Next, rollout of the statement begins. An internal publication program and inclusion of the statement in Associate orientation must be undertaken. Supervisors should give their staffs their own personal interpretation: "In our department, Respect means . . ." The concept is so simple and powerful that employees grasp it right away. The message to managers and Associates that accompanies presentation of the values must include the following points:

- The values statement supersedes all policy and practice. It is the most important guide in what we do.
- When you're not sure what to do in a situation, refer to the values and use your common sense. If what you're about to do fits the values, go ahead. If it doesn't, don't do it under any circumstances.
- The values statement is a hunting license that empowers all of us. If you see anything that needs changing because it doesn't fit the values, go ahead and change it yourself, turn in a suggestion, form a DIG, or report it to your supervisor. Anything that doesn't fit with the values is to be changed.
- The values are the basis by which your performance will be evaluated. You must live the values or you do not belong here.

One hospital president was walking down a hallway shortly after the rollout of the values statement in his organization when he saw one of the housekeeping staff. She had taped the Credo to the side of her supply cart, and he paused to ask what she thought of it. She responded, "Well, I read it first thing in the morning to help get me focused on what I'm supposed to be doing today. And when I'm having a bad day, I reread it to help me remember why I'm so important here. You know, if you think about it, this is really what life is all about." As the president proceeded down the hall he couldn't help but exclaim, "It's working!"

A terrible example of what not to do occurred in a large Chicago teaching hospital after they created a splendid values statement. Although they were caught up in its beauty and developed a wonderfully slick set of pamphlets, they failed to tie it into systems, and managers were not committed to it. Executives thought they were contributing something in the isolation of their paneled offices, but it didn't mean anything to the people cleaning the floors; it didn't serve as a prod to change. Like so many other failed agendas, it skated across the surface of the organization, another case of showcasing over substance. In change management, one learns not to squander these opportunities.

Values "Writ Large"

In addition to people in top management, human resources, and education, staff in public relations and marketing should be involved in the internal rollout campaign of the new values statement. It is essential to view the internal market as most important in communicating the values statement. Give concerted effort to the program. Staging significant events, writing internal media coverage, distributing posters, and holding special meetings are ideas that will pay off in the external market as Associates spread the word in the community.

There will be a natural inclination on the part of some Associates to wonder whether this is just another management gimmick, another here-it-comes, there-it-goes program. Don't minimize the communication task that must be accomplished. Nor should management think that simply announcing the program is going to be sufficient. There will be some key tests and key issues that the values statement must face; only then will staff begin to believe in it.

Enforcing Values

If the values are not going to be absolutely required, if management is not prepared to pay the price to enforce them, then organizational renewal should not be undertaken. "Put your money where your mouth is" is a test statement in our culture, as is "Put up or shut up." If you're not prepared to walk the walk, don't talk the talk.

For example, once you enunciate the respect value, the next incident of staff abuse by a physician will have to be tackled head-on. Management will have no choice but to deal with it, since publication of the values statement puts management out on a limb. The good news is that management decisions that are unpopular with abusers of the organization will no longer be considered personally directed. It is possible to say, "Dr. Jensen, I'm sorry I have to pull your privileges, but the values statement subscribed to by the entire management team and approved by the board, which has more weight than medical staff bylaws, requires me to take this action." Service, respect, excellence, and the other enunciated values become absolute requirements of all participants in the organization.

Action Plan for Managing Change

As each leader, executive, manager, or supervisor considers how to implement renewal changes in his or her area of responsibility, it's helpful to think things through carefully. The next step is to create a specific action plan to manage the change for which each person is responsible. The following list of questions will allow you to take inventory to ensure that all of the major elements of change management have been covered in your thought process. Use these proven questions to test the adequacy of your preparation. Put a star beside items you need to consider or do something about as part of your change plan.

Play into the Change Formula
1. Increase *dissatisfaction* over the present way of doing things among sponsors or other affected groups.
2. Refine the *model*. Make it simpler, more comprehensive, easier to understand, and slicker.
3. Improve *processing* by:
    *   Establishing a communication plan
    *   Talking with informal group leaders
    *   Talking with employees singly
    *   Talking with employees in group meetings
    *   Setting up employee work groups to work on pieces of the project
    *   Accepting workable employee suggestions
    *   Announcing the change as far in advance as possible

4. Assess the total situation in terms of both planning and implementation.

Control Situational Factors
1. Gain understanding of the history operating in this situation.
2. Factor the existing organizational culture into the plan.
3. Assess the timing and appropriateness of the change given the amount of past change the target population has had to deal with and the realities of the present situation.
4. Add to or strengthen the list of driving forces.
5. Shorten or weaken the list of restraining forces.
6. Add to the list of benefits. Find additional values to recommend the change (rewards, status, responsibility, achievement, autonomy, working relationships, etc.).
7. Reduce the lists of costs or their penalty.
8. Couple an unpopular change with a popular one or add a sweetener.
9. Gain the acceptance and respect of others as the change leader.
10. Ask whether it will be possible for the change leader to sustain the physical, intellectual, and emotional energy required.

Design the Work Plan
1. Correctly estimate the time and resources needed to support the change effort (everything takes longer, is harder, and costs more than you think). Are there built-in time buffers or extra budget allowances in case of delay or overruns?
2. Assess the personal risks and the risks to key political supporters.
3. Assess the organizational risks.
4. Define your fundamental commitments and redefine what needs changing.
5. Specify the process, the model, and the time line.
6. Do the legitimate work of worrying and help others deal with their worries by engaging in joint planning (as opposed to relying on the rumor mill).

7. Be decisive about small commonsense issues to cut against the grain of abounding uncertainty.
8. Prepare for the fact that more work than can possibly be anticipated will be required.

Be Politically Sensitive
1. Build coalitions and find support players to back the change effort.
2. Determine whether the timing is right.
3. Determine whether this is the right opportunity to go for broke or whether change will have to be implemented incrementally.
4. Listen carefully to all constituencies.
5. Ask whether you have been realistic or have bitten off more than you can chew.
6. Support people's personal planning and agendas in addition to planning for the project.
7. Acknowledge factional interests that merit consideration in order to diminish others' exaggerated bargaining positions.
8. Pave the road toward the goal to make it as smooth as possible.
9. Remember that managing change requires more emphasis on processing than on model building.
10. Remember that people need support from their supervisors and people-centered, not task-centered, leadership in order to master change.

Sequencing Organizational Change

Table 9.1 shows the sequence of organizational change that my Associates and I have developed over the last decade in working with many hospitals. (From here on, I will sometimes use *we* or *our* to denote the work of our consulting team. I will revert to first person when it is my personal observation.) This change sequence is derived from research and field experience. As a road map it works well in anticipating and planning for most of

Table 9.1. Sequencing Organizational Change.

Wave	Phase	Objective
Preparation (3 months)	Organizational change diagnostics	Assess readiness and fit
	Building executive commitment and consensus	Develop change action plan
	Strategically focusing the business	Link change and business objectives
	Planning and coordination	Establish support elements
	Organizational design and structure	Consolidate and collapse structure
Implementation (12 months)	Intensive management development	Build leadership team
	Implementing organizational renewal recommendations	Change organizational culture
	Cascading organizational change	Penetrate the organization
	Involving medical staff and board	Involve key stakeholders
	Measuring baseline and outcome	Assess improvement, targets, and progress
Acceleration (9 months)	Retargeting	Drive business results
	Institutionalizing change systems and culture	Solidify organization development gains
	Unleashing power of customer and innovation	Improve organization's responsiveness
	Intensifying systems improvement	Improve decision making, speed
	Deepening development of management and associate	Build on management strengths
	Driving change with evaluation and rewards	Better focus performance
	Revisiting structural design	Further improve accountability

the major change events, but it still allows for variation, customizing, and unanticipated crisis-handling capability. The entire process takes about two years, with the majority of the transformation being accomplished in fifteen months.

The Preparation Wave

In the preparation phase the organization is gearing up, doing enough diagnostic work to be sure that everyone involved understands the situation, developing the work plan, and making assignments. It is a time of great anticipation and hope, and for some it is also a time of high anxiety. While much will be expected of the change effort, effective executives will sometimes dampen expectations, preferring to underpromise and overdeliver.

The president may be heavily involved in answering questions from the board and physicians. This is the phase when executives have to get their act together. All of the basic assumptions about how the organization operates, how it's structured, and how the change can be dealt with become topics of numerous discussions. Chapter Ten will discuss the preparation wave in more detail.

The Implementation Wave

The second wave is a rapid yet thorough implementation of the renewal effort. This requires a detailed set of plans and operating guides that are controlled by the organization, with some outside coaching from a consultant. The main features of the implementation strategy are an intensive management development process to equip managers with the skills and techniques they need for their much expanded role in the New American Hospital and a simultaneous attack on hundreds of defects in the functioning of the organization. This latter part of the strategy is the true focus of the organization's renewal effort; it creates a hospital that produces excellent results through wide-scale involvement of Associates in problem-solving groups.

During this year, the pace of change moves from quick to

fast to frenetic. Dozens of tasks, projects, and work items are being completed each day. A change reaction begins to build, and the staff thrives on creative chaos. Chapter Eleven provides a highly detailed approach we have evolved over the last decade while working on hospital revitalization.

The Acceleration Wave

While approximately 75 percent of the change work is accomplished during the first two waves, the acceleration period is essential to make the changes stick. In this period, the gains that have been made thus far are consolidated and refined. This is also a time to institutionalize these changes so that the organization doesn't slip back, a common regression problem that undermines much organization development work. Now, also, managers who have been responsible for the change effort are rotated and the reward systems are refreshed—all changes that will recharge the driving forces for the project.

At this point the organization begins to swagger, filled with pride over its accomplishments. Accelerating the change process becomes vital so that people are rechallenged and not allowed to rest on their laurels. Chapter Twelve provides a more detailed view of where change programs run into difficulty, how these problems can be avoided or managed, and how to do the positive work of accelerating and consolidating change.

Note

1. The change management formula was authored by Michael Beer at Harvard University Graduate School of Business; the discussion comes from a number of presentations I was privileged to hear. Specific reference is given to M. Beer, *Organization Development: Its Nature, Origins, and Prospects* (Santa Monica, Calif.: Goodyear Press, 1980).

10

Preparing
for Transformation

Be Prepared.
— Boy Scouts of America

"Plan ahead" is more than just good advice; it's essential when contemplating making organization-wide changes that will affect nearly every aspect of the way Customers are dealt with, Associates are utilized, and management performs its work. Like a good physician, diagnosis comes before prescription, and the chapter opens with a discussion of organizational change diagnostics. Table 10.1 describes how the discussion moves on to building executive commitment, without which the change program would fail.

Proper management of the change program is not sufficient if other aspects of the organization's needs must also be attended to in terms of strategically focusing the business. The most critical task, and the one that starts things rolling, is to assemble the change team that will handle the planning and

Table 10.1. Preparation Wave.

Phase	Objective
Organizational change diagnostics	Assess readiness and fit
Executive commitment and consensus building	Develop change action plan
Strategically focus the business	Link change and business objectives
Planning and coordination	Establish support elements
Organizational design and structure	Consolidate and collapse structure

coordination of the project. Finally, a brief reference is made to the need to have an initial look at organizational structure insofar as it affects the ability to carry out the change action plan. In practice, it takes about three months of concentrated effort to carry out these tasks.

Diagnosing the Change Situation

Whether you are acting as a newly assigned executive in a takeover situation or a revitalizing executive who is transforming the organization, it's important to get a good fix on where the strengths and weaknesses, needs and opportunities, lie within the organization. Organizational diagnostics help assure that change is directed in an effective manner in terms of cost and effort. A common management failing is undertaking change on a piecemeal basis, often without understanding the complexity of the situation or the interrelatedness of the pieces. A physician would not prescribe without diagnosis and neither must the leader of the modern health care organization. At the same time, successful leaders start changing things before all the diagnostics are in—it's all right to do the obvious. Diagnostics are never used as a stall or a reason not to act.

Determining Change Readiness

Nothing is more threatening to an executive's career than a good change program implemented at the wrong time or under the wrong conditions. Assessing an organization's readiness for change helps ensure that the conditions are right and the timing is appropriate. I have developed an Organizational Performance and Readiness Assessment instrument to use as a quick measure in assessing whether these conditions are present. Change readiness is more likely to be present when there are a number of organizational failings, and when questions concerning executive support and political climate are rated positively. Some sample questions follow:[1]

1. Improvement needs
   - Customer satisfaction: Do you understand in detail your customer's expectations regarding your products and services?
   - Productivity: Does the organization meet its production schedules? Is work done on time?
   - People strength: Are the people in your organization doing the best work that they are capable of doing and is it acceptable?
2. Executive support
   - Is the CEO or executive in charge committed to changing things in the organization? Is he or she dissatisfied with things as they are?
3. Political climate
   - In the clinches when conflict occurs, do managers find themselves supported rather than compromised?

Additional questions are asked in areas of clarity of values, assessment of career management and performance, the history of management development, and whether the organization has a management system, organizational structure change needs, and change management procedures. For some organizations, the diagnostic phase may be an acute need, requiring a thorough research protocol. For most, the need is not as severe. As a rule, do enough assessment to understand the situation, but don't overspend scarce organizational resources on research that would be better spent on programmatic change.

Readiness is a composite of many things. There is no single profile of the ready organization. To some degree executives know it when they see it. They have a sense of what's needed and the appropriate time to do it. As a consultant, I know that a call from a client is an indication of some degree of organizational readiness and the client's concern about a number of problems. Readiness is also indicated if managerial KRAs or organizational outcomes are deficient, power blocs are upset, employees are angry, or the market is deserting the organization.

Determining that an organization is in a state of readiness

does not allow you to say that a change effort will be successful. All that can be said is that conditions look favorable, or that change is needed. People's minds may be more open to new thinking now, or other factors may have come together that favor the attempt.

The CEO and Change Readiness

The major indicator of readiness is the CEO. From my experience there seems to be a psychographic profile of the CEO who undertakes major organizational change. Nearly all CEOs retaining me to perform organizational change work are between the ages of thirty-five and fifty, generally have been with the organization less than five years, and have been CEO less than two years (most less than one year). Therefore, the typical picture of the change leader is that of a younger executive, new to the organization, and new to the top management spot. Being new in their position, these CEOs have nothing to defend. Being new to the organization, they've had other experiences and other points of view and don't buy into the organizational group-think that prevails. Being young, they have the physical and psychological energy needed to carry the work forward. Stating the reverse hypothesis, older executives may be too tired or too comfortable with the status quo to be able to challenge the patterns of practice they created over the years. There are, however, notable exceptions.

I will never forget the sixty-two-year-old hospital CEO who had been in charge of his hospital for thirty years. Nearly all aspects of its operation had come from his decision making. I told him of my experience that change usually requires a younger person, and I queried his ability to take the project forward. His response was instructive: "I have three more years until retirement. This is the time in which we must change the hospital world, and I intend to make this last major program my monument." He further explained that undertaking this program was like Ronald Reagan negotiating arms reductions with Mikhail Gorbachev. "If a liberal Democrat had undertaken it, it might have been politically suspect. Similarly, my credentials as a member of the establishment allow me to criticize any past decisions and people will buy it." I'd call that a sign of organizational change readiness, wouldn't you? The transition process proved to be somewhat difficult for this senior executive, but he pulled it off.

Assessing the Executive Team

The vice presidential layer and certain key directors will be critical to the change plan. Lose no time in determining whether they have the horsepower to implement the plan. From a practical standpoint, the top executive will succeed or fail by how well these folks do. There is little to be gained by waiting for problems to surface.

If you're in a turnaround situation, you need to ask difficult questions: Should the executive group that stifled this organization remain? If I were looking for a replacement, would I hire this person for the job? This is a time for mental toughness. *The best predictor of an executive's future track record is his or her past track record.* If these people haven't been winners in the past, are you ready to bet your career and organization on them?

It must also be said that good executives are often tarred by the programs and decisions of a past leader. It's possible that under new leadership they might be substantially better players. In sports, many ball players do terribly on one team, get traded, and wind up going to the Hall of Fame. The difference lies in the quality of coaching they receive. How good are the executives, and how good could they be with the right leadership?

Regardless of whether the CEO is working with a stable team of known winners or taking over a troubled organization, move rapidly to remove obstacles reported by the seconds- and thirds-in-command. Free them up to do all that they can do. This maximizes their chance of succeeding and removes the stones under which people hide. If they then don't perform, the complaints were just excuses for them not to perform.

Assessing the Management Team

If executives are considered the field generals, then middle managers are the captains and lieutenants who must carry the brunt of the battle. They must be men and women of courage and vision, who are committed to the plan and to the many changes that are about to take place. Are the right people on the battlefield? Do they have what it takes?

Move quickly, using reports from vice presidents and your own interviews with middle managers, to determine whether talent and conviction are present or can be sparked. Without demoralizing or terrorizing those who will support you, get rid of those who can't or don't want to get the job done. Don't go into battle with the walking wounded and the walking dead and the on-the-job retirees.

Studies of organizations undergoing massive change show that most resistance does not develop at Associate levels but in the ranks of middle and upper management. Often these people have the most to lose from changing the status quo. In the major organization development projects I've been involved with, the number of managers who were eventually replaced amounted to 5 to 25 percent of the group, usually in the low end of that range. Housecleaning was done over time, sometimes not until peers voiced loud dissatisfaction with those who were not adopting the emerging group norms.

As with the executives, have the middle managers create a list of obstacles they would like to see removed, and identify what else they may need in order to enter the fray on your behalf. This initial list will get a lot longer and more specific as the organizational revolution gets under way, so keep asking this question.

Assessing Associates' Morale

It's essential to know Associates' feelings and thoughts regarding the organization. The success of the entire change effort depends on them. If a full opinion study is not possible before kicking off the change process, an easy way to determine the human issues is to meet with several groups of Associates. Measuring employee morale just prior to, or shortly after, the onset of a major organization development effort accomplishes several objectives.

First, Associate opinion surveys provide a baseline against which changes in the organization can be gauged. When the survey is rerun twelve to eighteen months later, management will be able to determine whether they are winning the battle for the hearts and minds of Associates.

Second, measuring the human climate always brings to light the major issues and hundreds of specific problems that expose any Achilles' heel the organization may have. This bad news helps to provide *dissatisfaction energy*, which is useful in driving change forward. Rather than being the only one to provide this needed mobilizing energy, the executive in charge of the change program is now able to speak on behalf of the entire work force, a tremendously powerful assist! The array of problems becomes a justification for major organizational change. In my experience, doing one of these surveys is like setting off an atom bomb.

Similarly, the positive changes resulting from opinion surveys create a momentum made up of good change vibrations within the organization. Large organization development changes can then hitch a ride on this momentum in a kind of piggyback phenomenon.

Assessing Unmet Market and Customer Needs

Customers' needs and their perception of the hospital should be included in assessing the human organization. Customers are part of the hospital, not just recipients of what it does. Organization development is not achieved in a vacuum with no relation to the external operating environment. Just as unanswered Associate needs provide a source of dissatisfaction energy, so, too, do unmet Customer needs, which can be used as a driving force to change internal operations.

As one hospital president began his overall change effort, he established Committees of Excellence comprised of major Customer segments. These groups quickly helped physicians and department heads to understand why change was needed. The groups identified a full array of unmet needs, unanswered problems, poor service responses, and unnecessary administrative tangles. Wave after wave of recommendations bombarded various departments with the clear message to change.

Thus the hospital president, instead of having to personally persuade managers, used Customer energy to force change.

By identifying Customer needs the hospital can improve services, operate in a more profitable way, and attract a greater market share. The skillful change executive is always looking for ways to use problems in one area to drive solutions in another. Unhappy Customers represent both change readiness and change energy.

Assessing Cultural Impacts

Corporate culture can be described as "the way we do things around here," the combined total of the official and unofficial norms that guide behavior, and the simple standards of measurement and rules of thumb that people use to know when they are on target. All societies, tribes, nations, and organizations have a culture that guides members in their behavior, the decisions they make, and the risks they're willing to take. Understanding the limits and strengths of that culture is essential in making wide-scale change.

For the executive leading organizational change, I recommend a reasoned assessment of how the proposed change might have impacts on the culture. Organizational renewal may be more difficult to accomplish in an organization that is very cautious, risk averse, highly authoritarian, and with religious overseers, than it would be in a Southern California hospital where all the executives have been to consciousness-raising seminars and come to work in Hawaiian shirts! But, surprisingly, sometimes just the opposite is true.

Not only should the difficulty of change be assessed, but also how rapidly it can be achieved given the political situation. What is it possible to do in this situation? How should this particular culture be addressed? What cultural strengths can be used to drive change? Another important question is how a successful series of changes will affect the culture. Will they strengthen its good parts? Will they eliminate or weaken its bad parts? Will the debate and the pain that is caused be beneficial? Even if it's possible to accomplish this change, is it the right thing to do? We don't make change in a vacuum. We make it in the context of who we are and where we've come from as an organization.

Building Executive Commitment

Once the president decides to undertake organizational change, the political processes needed to build support for the effort can be started. This calls for a lot of talking and even arm twisting to make sure that all parties are on board. The essential groups that presidents are most concerned with are the executive team, the board, and physicians.

Taking the Blood Oath

Successful change executives hold a Leadership Advance (no more management retreats!) with their vice presidents. An agenda is constructed to get at the major issues that organizational transformation creates. Each participant airs his or her concerns about the change program. The best sessions are often those with heated exchanges and full and open discussions. Out of disagreement comes truth. One by one, executives are asked to declare themselves. A declaration of commitment is signed, which will be published throughout the house. People are asked to go on record and to risk embarrassment if they don't deliver.

In my approach I ask the executives as a team to sign the statement, "We the Leadership Team of [name of hospital] commit ourselves to organizational excellence and will accept nothing less." Wording changes are acceptable as long as they do not water down the statement to "We'll try to be more excellent" or drop the promise to "accept nothing less." I have found that it's important not to let the group think that if you soften the wording, the statement will carry the same weight, and I dismiss any such efforts.

While this may seem to be only a silly symbol, unless the executives are prepared to sign and commit to excellence, I refuse any further part in the organization development effort. I do this to underscore the fact that decisions come before programs, not the other way around. I usually do this exercise early on the first day. Too often, hospital teams talk endlessly and dance around issues. Unless people are willing to put their name on the line and state that they're not going to accept anything less than excellence, all you've got is . . . nothing.

Later this blood oath is duplicated and posted on executive walls in type large enough to be read from across the room. It begins to raise questions in the minds of the managers and Associates who see it. As the management team is brought into the process, they are also allowed to sign the statement. So the document is used as a seed to get discussion and behavior rolling.

There are always some people who will go along verbally but who do not truly support the change. Don't worry about it. The president has done the job of trying to communicate what is expected. If those who eat at the table do not enjoy the feast, let them dine out in the future.

Identifying Thought Leaders

It's necessary to gain political support among all of the hospital's constituencies. This includes the board, physicians, various community groups, and other persons of influence such as business leaders. A good strategy is to start with thought leaders and get them on board. In one client intervention, the eight "Good Guys," physicians who were highly influential in their specialties, were invited by the chairman of the medical staff to attend an evening dinner. For three hours we discussed the change effort that was under way, why it was important, and what other hospitals were doing. The physicians were able to express their thoughts and give good counsel. Not all of them were totally convinced, but the doubters had their criticisms muted.

It is important to examine the various political blocs within the system. How good is the hospital's relationship with the medical staff? Where does the board stand? How about unions? Are the middle managers with you? Within each of these groups, who are the key players and thought leaders as opposed to those who are simply members of the group? Who will be for you, against you, or neutral to your positions? What issues will be important? What tradeoffs will you have to offer in order to gain support? How can you start people thinking through the issues so that they wind up in your camp? How can enemies of the change program be neutralized or overcome?

These power blocs and their agendas can be very helpful in driving change, particularly if they can see a connection between your program and some of the things they're trying to achieve for themselves. In the case of most hospitals, the senior power group's interests are clearly served by the New American Hospital model that emphasizes Customer service, no-excuse performance responsibility, openness to innovation, and better conflict management.

What About the Doctors and the Board?

My experience is that physicians as a group have never been an obstacle to an organizational excellence campaign. There may be some confusion at the outset about what the change represents, along with cynical doubts that anything of substance will result. The savvy executive spends quite a bit of time communicating with physicians, even putting them on the managers' newsletter distribution list or inviting them to sit in on management development sessions. As for the cynicism, achieve some results and it will take care of itself.

Physicians often wonder whether the change program will affect their business interests. The answer is yes. As the hospital builds its business, it also builds the physician's business. Invite doctors to attend or chair one of the problem-solving groups; give them a piece of the action.

Board members primarily ask: "Will this increase risk? Will it increase the hospital's stature?" Renewal reduces risks because the organization begins to deal with long-standing problem situations. Over time, as the organization dramatically improves, risk decreases, and as the organization becomes known for its superiority, its stature increases. Respond to the questions the board clearly wants answered. They often are curious about the mechanics of the renewal process and what the experience of other places has been. Again, follow the prescriptions of communication and participation.

Strategic Business Focus

Going forward with the new management approaches of the New American Hospital is not all that is necessary to win. In addition to following the management prescriptions in this book, it's necessary to make smart financial moves, market intelligently, protect physician relationships, and build new community coalitions. The business needs to sharpen its external focus while it is undergoing internal revitalization.

While this is not a text on competitive strategy, keep the importance of that art in mind when considering organizational change. If competitors are doing smarter things in the marketplace, while your market share is declining, it is doubtful that your superior organizational design will impress the board. Staying at least even with your competitors during the transition process is necessary to avoid jeopardizing the change program. The basic marketing rules apply. Follow them, gain market success, install the organization development work, and succeed over the competition! For example, ask if you are doing the following things:

- Divesting declining or low-revenue businesses
- Selling services directly to consumers or the industry
- Identifying growth markets and services and establishing dominant positions
- Considering taking over losing hospitals or services to build market share
- Targeting serviceable Customer segments
- Identifying market niches where defensible positions can be staked out
- Considering investing in new biotechnology, such as becoming a genetics center
- Financing changes out of profits to avoid debt

- Financing changes through for-profit restructuring to gain access to capital
- Considering joint ventures to reduce risk
- Achieving profitability, not market share, sales, or occupancy
- Setting a goal of having 25 percent of revenue come from services less than five years old

From the perspective of organizational transformation, it's wonderful to hear of new market successes and added services when you're returning tired from your third DIG meeting of the week! Nothing succeeds like success, and better external targeting of the market can be a potent asset in building the New American Hospital. But knowing what the competition is doing, and outflanking and outperforming them, isn't the whole story. Too many hospitals still fall into the old pattern of duplicating what other hospitals across town are doing—if the others get a lithotripter, you get a lithotripter. Managing for excellence doesn't start with what the competition is doing, but with what the Customer needs and with your own vision of what excellence will require. The New American Hospital is less concerned with keeping up with the Joneses than it is with outinnovating and outserving them. Accept that you're no longer in a horse race with these people. Get off the track they're on and seek your own path. Let others imitate you, if they can. Learn to become an original.

Planning and Coordination

Change agents are needed to carry out executive direction of the transformation. Theoretically, this could be done by the line organization, but they are already busy with other things, like running the hospital! Also, the existing line structure is often too entrenched with too many reasons to defend the status quo.

Another avenue might be to add an organization development specialist to the staff. Field experience suggests that while these folks have much to offer, they often lack a change mandate and political clout. The worst are those who bog down, redrawing the organizational chart, making studies, and trying to sell piecemeal applications.

What's needed is something akin to George Patton and the Third Army, a force that can take off and go after prime targets without too much other baggage. This means setting up new power groups to handle the task and using them to create a detailed plan. What follows is a description of such an approach to the development of a tactical plan for change.

Establishing New Groups to Handle Renewal

Nearly all approaches to leading wide-scale change set up a steering group and other support elements to look after pieces of the project. The following description is our particular approach to this need. Less important than how the organizing is done is the fact that issues are effectively managed.

Management Action Council (MAC). The MAC is a middle-management group of five to seven of the brightest and most respected managers, who are so indispensable that they probably can't be spared! The busiest people are often the ones you need most. They act as a representative group for all managers and are in charge of the overall implementation of the plan. The chairperson of the MAC reports directly to the president.

The group steers the various project action teams, sells upward to executives, and actively brokers the overall change effort. Think of them as a special commando team, a group that spins out dozens of other management and Associate change groups. The MAC also helps implement new systems such as the idea engine and Customer service strategy. The MAC carries out a detailed checklist of items developed for the overall renewal effort, issues special assignments to such departments as Finance and Human Resources to develop new pieces of the plan, and monitors how well each manager is doing. The advantage of such an approach is that it bypasses the existing line structure and makes the change program one that is driven by the managers—it becomes their program.

Socialization Action Council (SAC). The SAC is a small group of "party animals" who do the unbelievable task of putting on an entire series of social events over the period of organizational change. Following the rule that excellent teams are those that work hard and play hard, the SAC makes sure that people party hearty. Initially their focus is on the management team, encouraging them and helping them with their distress during the difficult days of organizational change. Later, as the achievements begin to roll in, the added function of celebration for work well done begins to flower. Eventually the SAC cascades down to the Associate level where it becomes the mother of all SACs, spinning off new SAC groups that sponsor even more wide-scale social activity. The SAC chairperson is a member of the MAC.

Communication Action Council (CAC). The CAC publicizes what the program of change is all about and posts all completed pieces of the change program, including all project completions, on a Victory Scoreboard. Their task is to provide an intensive internal marketing campaign to all Associates to convince them that the changes are for the benefit of the organization. The CAC chairperson is also a member of the MAC.

The CAC counteracts the confusion created by change and sends the change drumbeat throughout the organization. It creates newsletters, places daily Change-Grams on cafeteria tables, and organizes departmental Communication Centers and other media blitz efforts. One hospital devoted fully half of its marketing department resources to the CAC. In time its Associates became extremely effective voices in the community, full of pride in what their hospital had become. It is absolutely essential that people come to believe in the New American Hospital, and belief in it requires this intense communication effort.

Executive Vision Council. This is a group of executives and the MAC. It meets at least weekly, often twice a week during the start-up phase. Its key issues are problems concerning the change effort. It does not meet to get executive approvals. The MAC makes most of the change decisions, but it refers major policy questions to Executive Vision. Because it isn't problem-focused, Executive Vision looks at the overall direction and strategy and the larger hopes and dreams for the change effort.

This meeting is the place in which executive egos are sensitized as they receive feedback on deficiencies no one had the courage to tell them about before!

Special Project Assignees. A number of other managers and departments are players during the preparation wave. Over sixty projects are assembled prior to the program and are handled by making assignments to individual managers. Following are sample assignments:

- Create productivity charts: Industrial engineer or Accounting
- Presentation on "What I Like to See in a Proposal": President/CEO
- Presentation on "Disciplinary Procedures": Human Resources
- Redesign organizational structure, streamline approvals: President/CEO
- Abolish obsolete financial management practices: Chief financial officer
- Tie management pay to Customer and Staff evaluations: Human Resources
- Create "Manager's Survival Guide": President/CEO
- Recognize KRA achievements: MAC
- Identify resources for DIG improvements: Chief financial officer
- Update organizational literature to reflect changes in language: CAC
- Create a values-centered guide for all Associates: MAC
- Provide DIG process training for Associates: Education and Training

Consultants. Should an organization desiring organizational renewal do it on its own or get outside help? For most hospitals the answer is to go to the outside. If this is done it's imperative that internal change agents such as those listed above are also used; otherwise the whole concept of listening to the voices inside is stifled.

The outside resource person can supply an already developed model and the lessons it has taught. A key to success is when the consultant's model is open-ended and therefore adaptable to the needs of the organization. In addition, internal management must be the implementors of the program; the organization must not become dependent on the consultant at this critical point, but should use the consultant to save time, rapidly accelerate the change, and verify that key elements are not overlooked. The consultant acts with a mandate, functions very much like a de facto vice president in charge of change, and reports directly to the president. To fulfill this role correctly, he or she must lead the organization into deep water, but not drown it; push it, but not shove it to the point of resistance; be helpful, but not do the work that the organization must do for itself.

Creating a Change Action Plan

The elements of the action plan and the support materials needed to carry it out include:

1. A picture of the New American Hospital. What specific elements do we want to build into the way we do things? What will the hospital look like? How will it behave? What pieces of work will have to be done to pull it off? Much of that content is represented in this book.
2. A Gantt chart to specify what work will be done, when, and by whom.
3. Support guides for the MAC, SAC, and CAC that give them operational procedures, specify the do's and don't's of their role, and supply forms and other details necessary to carry out their duties.
4. Instructions for each special assignment.
5. A management development plan, schedule of events, and lists of assignments for each session.
6. An Executive Guide to help officers understand their new role and how to perform it. This is a needed structural piece to walk them into the new behaviors required of them.

7. A master Administrative Guide that spells out how all of these pieces interrelate and how change should be carried out.

Organizing these pieces at the outset will give you much greater control over what is always a daunting and confusing project. Like everything else of significance, God is in the details.

Rethinking the Organizational Structure

The organizational structure of the old hospital is incompatible with the relationships, patterns of work accomplishment, Customer needs, and communication requirements called for in the New American Hospital. The preparation wave may not be the best time to launch all the structural changes that are needed, but some are worth doing. For those that are not timely, it's a good idea to start making preliminary judgments about what might need to be done. The next good time window for making adjustments is at the end of the second, or implementation, wave. (See Chapter Seven for a further discussion on reorganization options.)

Note

1. Adapted from C. Sherman, Organization Performance and Readiness Assessment (Inverness, Ill.: Management House).

11

Implementing the Renewal Strategy

Only great battles produce great results. . . . Many assume
that half efforts can be effective. A small jump is easier than a
large one, but no one wishing to cross a wide ditch would
cross half of it first.
— Baron Karl von Clausewitz
On War[1]
(His strategy destroyed Napoleon's
army in the Russian winter.)

This chapter details how the implementation wave is carried out.
As such it illustrates one approach to making the major changes
required for organizational renewal. In this approach, a dual
track is followed to organizational change — simultaneously participating in intensive management development and, with a
short time lag, concurrently implementing recommendations
for organizational renewal. The objective of the former is to
create changes in management behavior, and of the latter to
accomplish organizational change. The discussion then moves
to the question of how to cascade organizational change, in
terms of both downward participation to Associates and out-
ward to the medical staff and the board, as well as to increase
actual penetration of change into the organization. Finally, the
chapter looks at the important question of baseline and outcome measurements to ensure that the change program has
worked, and return-on-investment calculation to ensure that it
has been cost-effective.

Table 11.1 shows the phases of the implementation wave.
Having politically prepared the organization and put together
the change plan and coordination pieces, the leadership team is
now ready to unleash the pent-up human energy within the

Table 11.1. Implementation Wave.

Phase	Objective
Intensive management development	Build leadership team
Implement organizational renewal recommendations	Change the organization and its systems of managing
Cascade organizational change	Penetrate the organization
Involve medical staff and board	Involve key stakeholders
Measure baselines and outcomes	Assess improvement targets and progress

organization. The change model described here is based on my experience in doing hospital transformations since 1980. This model, called The Uncommon Leader, contains a number of common core elements that other organization development practitioners and I have found to work. Examine the model critically to see if it is appropriate and tolerable to your organization. Beyond the question of the adequacy of the change program is the question of the organization's ability to execute and utilize such a program.

At the beginning of renewal, executives know that the business environment requires the hospital to change, but the exact picture of what the new organization should look like is not clear. There is always some ambiguity and fuzziness about how the program of action should be pursued, and what the end result will be. The goal of the intervention is to create a new and more effectively functioning organization.

A clear necessity in undertaking implementation is to relate the program design, timing, sequence, and change agents to the business realities at hand. If the workload of other hospital projects will be too great, unionization is imminent, or there's going to be a change in CEO, this might not be a wise undertaking, no matter how badly the organization might need it. There never is a perfect time to undertake such a change or a time when it will be easy; you must use your judgment about what the organization can realistically achieve.

Our approach to renewal combines building the manage-

ment team and at the same time making wide-scale organizational change. Management development is used to drive organization development. Intensive management development is
used by change-master executives to rapidly streamline operations and improve business results by creating a peak-
performing management team. This model provides systematic
education, operating systems, and group process mechanisms
to successfully complete the changeover. Experience has shown
that attempts to change organizations fail unless managers also
change. Improved organizations and improved management
come only from improved managers.

Undertaking Intensive Management Development

The general atmosphere among managers just before onset is
one of excitement. There is a general optimism and hope, even
when there has been a past history of program crashes. Managers report sensing that this effort will be more massive, seems
better organized, and holds more promise. In part this positive
expectation comes out of the extensive preparation and the
direct control managers have through the MAC, SAC, and CAC
coordination groups.

This positive feeling is offset by cynics, skeptics, and
doubters who've seen too many programs come and go. This
group acts as a helpful balancing mechanism, reminding others
of the magnitude of the challenge. This is a time of anxiety, some
fear, and many doubts. Managers are wondering if they will be
able to measure up, or if they will be embarrassed by the
program. Those who know they're incompetent sense the career
risk associated with the program. These fears are groundless as
long as people do the work, learn the lessons, and change their
behavior.

Development of the management team combines formal
classroom work with on-the-job experiences to achieve the
following:

*   Empowering managers to handle operations without execu-
    tive hand holding

- Increasing managerial skills and techniques
- Building team values and interdependency
- Improving the organization's performance and profitability
- Adding to risk taking and entrepreneurship
- Decentralizing decision making while maintaining executive control

A multiplicity of styles and philosophies are usually found in hospitals that compound the organization's problems. To be a winning team, it's important for managers to focus the change effort rather than fragmenting it. When management development sessions are allowed to function as a change arena, the classroom becomes a vehicle for rapid organizational change. There is safety in numbers—people speak their minds. And the group dynamics of a correctly organized and led hospital management team contain the answers the organization needs.

Selecting the Management Audience

In most hospitals, a majority of managers come from technical specialties and have little or no formal training in management. The organization that embarks on the development of its leaders is making a bet that their improved performance will affect functioning in the total organization. I have written elsewhere that it is inadvisable to think that training can do the whole job. If changes are contemplated that would create new managers or replace old ones, it is desirable to accomplish those changes prior to the start of the program. No matter how good the training effort is, it cannot make up for selecting mediocre managers.

Under previous patterns of organizational leadership, the typical hierarchical control model was followed. This created a passive, dependent management group, conditioned to wait for orders instead of creating initiatives. This trained inertia will have to be broken and a new responsive pattern inserted into the culture. If the natural resistance to change that can be expected from this key group cannot be overcome, or if there is just not enough intellectual and emotional capability to pull things through, then the program will be in jeopardy. These problems can be dealt with if there is a vigilant executive group willing to take action and a skilled classroom presenter who can deal with the symptoms of resistance.

The target audience needs to be identified, including the levels to be trained in the first wave, their numbers, and how operations will be handled while managers are in the classroom. As a practical matter, it is important not to invite participants who will not benefit from the training or who are not in agreement with the change direction. They retard classroom discussion. Not receiving a program invitation is a powerful message for them to rethink their career options.

Those who are invited attend an orientation meeting where the program's objectives and mechanics are laid out, with emphasis placed on the amount of work and change required of them as participants. The president should let people know that they can request a transfer out of management; some participants will select out of the process, an honest realization that they don't want the new role.

Program Objectives

A development effort of this caliber seeks to attain several key targets:

1. Build the business of the organization by creating a management force capable of achieving key business strategies and defeating competitors.
2. Increase the individual effectiveness and capabilities of the organization's managers as practitioners of their craft.
3. Increase team interplay and cooperation and find ways to break down interdepartmental rivalries and barriers. What is desired is high collaboration and low-competition interdependence subscribed to by independent-feeling managers.
4. Clarify and intensify the organization's values and mission.

5. Assist managers in coping with present change pressures and prepare them for future organizational demands.
6. Create a leadership cadre that is better prepared to help the organization attain quality, Customer satisfaction, productivity, profitability, and other key results.
7. Develop a self-renewing, viable, "loosened up" system that can organize in a variety of ways depending on the task.
8. Reach the point where decisions are made on the basis of information source, competence, and nearness to the problem rather than organizational position.

Rules to Run by

Before starting such an educational initiative, some clear rules must be followed to avoid later problems. Be careful when putting the pieces together and they won't come apart later on!

1. The change program concepts and mechanics must be approved in advance by the organization's CEO. Approval by the coordinating staff group alone is not sufficient since there may be political problems or resistance.
2. High-level executives' attendance at the program is required. There is no leadership other than that of example. The impact on managers who see their executives actively participating is powerful, and a greater bonding across management levels will result.
3. Attendance by all participants at all sessions is a requirement for program completion and graduation. Championship teams require attendance at spring training for all players, even the superstars. There are no shortcuts to excellence.
4. Management development will affect organizational change. During the program a number of management practices will be discussed and consensus votes for change will be sought from participants. The focus of the program is to create a new system of management within the organi-

zation. There should be expectations that when managers'
behavior changes, so will the organization.

5.   The expectation of participants is less that they should work
     harder, but that they change how they function. Since new
     managerial work roles have to be learned and old habits are
     not easily discarded, the workload for managers during the
     program is significant. Adoption of new management prac-
     tices will result in a net savings of time and in projects that
     are brought to conclusion with a minimum amount of slip/
     slide.

Building Managerial Muscle

Figure 11.1 shows how management development and organization development elements flow together. The program first
focuses on sharpening management-team performance. The
management development series centers around six two-day
presentation sessions. The educational sequence begins with a
presession study assignment; participants come to the classroom prepared and do not have to come up to speed in terms of
the discussion topic.

       Live presentations constitute the primary learning expe-
rience. It is essential that this be a practical, techniques oriented
experience in order to equip managers with the tools necessary
to do the change work. A serious mistake at this point would be
to have another boring day discussing simple principles or
academics that don't deal with the nitty-gritty problems of engaging in massive change.

       During the two-day seminars, a great deal of work is done
in small groups that relate the subject matter to actual changes
the organization needs to make; detailed assignments are given
about the tasks to be undertaken following the meeting. Each
session also contains time for socialization; it is followed two
weeks later by a film showcase. This one-two-three punch of
prereading, seminar attendance, and the film and assignments
reinforces the message for maximum impact. The seminar sessions are scheduled at eight-week intervals to allow completion

Figure 11.1. Organization Transformation via The The Uncommon Leader.

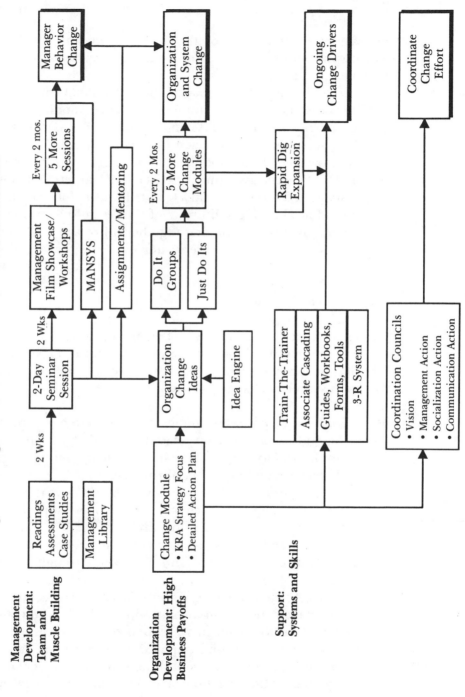

of assignments, readings for the next session, and the DIGs which spin out of every session. A sample agenda is given in Exhibit 11.1.

In addition to the management educational thrust, the MAC oversees the implementation of six change modules, each focused on one or more KRAs and continuing a specific and lengthy action plan of items that must accompany the insertion of new knowledge. Each modular action plan contains numerous Just Do It special assignments, a list of DIG targets that must be hit, suggested assignees, and a Gantt chart to plot timelines. These modules become subthrusts of the overall renewal program, emphasizing and pulling together all of the work that must be done around the core strategies of the revitalization effort.

Program Complements

Our experience is that a number of elements must be added to the management development sessions in order to make them effective for achieving behavioral change; we have not been able to obtain sufficient change without them.

- *Assignments.* Extensive assignments are given to participants at the end of each session related to needed changes the group decides to target. These lead to changes in managerial behavior and hospital performance.
- *Mentors.* To ensure that assignments are carried out, in-house mentors are assigned to each participant to review progress, and a completion record is forwarded to the MAC, which summarizes and reports to the president the behavior of any manager or executive who is not following through on the program.
- *MANSYS.* As the seminar series unrolls, various pieces of the new management system are introduced. Each segment is presented for the managers' acceptance. Following buy-in, the system's pieces become required management behavior.
- *Management library.* The establishment of the management library begins the insertion of variant management view-

points and concepts; these are needed to increase management literacy, avoid group-think, and prevent dependency on consultants.

- *Common texts and language.* To help build a common management language, several texts are required reading by all participants. From these and MANSYS emerge a set of core concepts that act as managerial unifiers.

Program Support Pieces

Management development changes managerial and organizational performance, but only under certain conditions. Classroom work alone is insufficient to change behavior. It is important to build in the systematic reinforcement and organizational change mechanisms necessary to make things different. In addition to the support pieces used in the preparation wave, I use the following during implementation:

- Executive Guide (sets out expectations for overall management)
- Participant and executive session assignments
- DIG Guide
- MANSYS, DIG, and values workshops
- Course Administration Guide
- Strategy manual and work plans for each change module
- Associate, Customer, and peer evaluation forms
- Idea Engine Guide
- Guides for the MAC, SAC, and CAC

Keep in mind that what is being described is only our model. Other approaches can be successful. Carefully thinking through what will help the program succeed can prevent a lot of problems. Some organizations will employ tools, processes, and program elements developed elsewhere, rather than reinventing the wheel or attempting change solely by in-house means. But when you use any outside program, recognize that it's a beginning platform from which your organization must evolve its own

Exhibit 11.1. Outline of Recommended Content.

Because the overriding concern is how to best affect organizational change, the management development (MD) content and series sequence are based on what will help managers affect the course of renewal.

Module I: "Profiles in Excellence"
MD Day 1: "Creating the New American Hospital"
Explains the need for the New American Hospital and gets confirmation from the management audience of the need to change. Identifies where the organization wants to go in its performance. Assesses the management team's commitment to creating organizational excellence and maps out the plan of action. A day of challenge and target identification.

MD Day 2: "Uncommon Leadership & Management Effectiveness"
Behaviors, practices, techniques, and beliefs that pay off in winning performance. A detailed profiling of each manager's present performance, and an action plan of how to manage work, time, people, decisions, and priorities. Introduction to the new management system, MANSYS.

OD Change Notes: The focus of this opening session is to create clear pictures of how winning organizations perform and what winning managers do to get results. The session serves to fire the imagination and to lift the sights of the leadership team. The first parts of the management system are introduced, along with the first recommendations for change from the management group. Here, as for all following modules, is introduced the action plan for this session's identified KRA targets.

Module II: "The Power of People"
MD Day 1: "Leading People to Growth & Contribution"
Tapping the sources of motivation in today's Associates and providing the leadership challenge. Describes how to get people's support through motivational management and achievement-reward systems.

MD Day 2: "From Losers to Winners: Transforming Problem People"
Not everyone belongs on a championship team. Shows how to get nonperformers out of the organization or help them come back to high-performance levels. Preparation of action plans for problem Associates.

OD Change Notes: This session focuses on people management questions, in terms of both obtaining better performances from good people and redirecting or controlling misfit behavior. This part of the program equips the team to do whatever housecleaning may be required on problem cases, and the organization should be prepared to back managers' recommendations in this area.

Module III: "Customers: The Reason for Being"
MD Day 1: "The Customer Is King"
Business success comes only from satisfied Customers. The team plans how to implement a complete Customer service strategy including satisfaction measurement, Customer empowerment, and approaches to letting the Customer teach you your business.

MD Day 2: "Accountability in Management"
Checking to see if tasks get done, and done right, with no excuses for nonperformance. Control is not a dirty word. Using aggressive leadership. Redeploying resources to solve problems instead of asking for more staff and more budget.

OD Change Notes: This session examines the central issues surrounding dynamic Customer service, the empowerment of the Customer, identification of unmet Customer needs, and creation of a year-long tactical plan for improvement. The session also reviews the implementation system and the need for cost management.

Module IV: "Risking for Greatness"
MD Day 1: "Managerial Muscle: Power and Persuasion"
Teaching how to be politic without being political. Selling ideas within the organization. Showing how to press for new approaches without being offensive. Explaining the use of proposal formats. Multiplying empowerment elements already under way.

MD Day 2: "Creativity and Controlling the Chaos of Change"
Change and innovation are thought of as essential for any organization's future. Dealing with resistance to change and using resistant energy in positive ways. Redefining conflict and using it for accomplishment. Instituting conflict management protocols.

OD Change Notes: Dealing with the informal political world and selling ideas in that world are the focus of this part of the program. It emboldens and encourages managers to take more initiative; executives are required to respond to support needs from the group that will grant them greater power to deal with the change and conflict affecting the organization.

Module V: "Quality, Speed, and Results"
MD Day 1: "Continuous Improvement: Saving Time, Money, & Effort"
At this point there has been enough cultural change to begin implementing work improvement systems. The focus is on problem solving and defining what the problem is and is not. The uses of data and measures are explored, and the key tests of Customer input and quality outcomes are used.

MD Day 2: "Power Tools, Methods, & Workable Solutions"
The focus is on the use of weighted decision-making matrices, trial implementations, basic industrial engineering, and work simplification procedures. The limited use of statistical sampling techniques is begun in selected areas. Teaching when and where to use tools in order to avoid common TQM failures in hospitals.

OD Change Notes: The system-improvement session provides more sophisticated problem-analysis tools. Our experience is that managers are better prepared for these tools after the experiential learning that occurs in small work groups during the early portion of the program. At this point Associates also should begin training in continuous improvement methods.

Module VI: "Unifying Team Performance"
MD Day 1: "Maximizing Productivity & Innovation"
Getting the work out. Improving organizational efficiency and conserving scarce resources while improving levels of quality. Specific action planning for both individual managers and the organization.

MD Day 2: "Building a Winning Team"
Discusses characteristics of effective teams and how they are formed. Examines current organizational needs and creates an opportunity to work on future game plans. Winning with the "heart of a champion."

OD Change Notes: The final segment of the program looks at how all the pieces of the puzzle have to fit together in order to get the work out and build greater team cohesion and family alliance. At this point the group critiques the change program and makes recommendations for the acceleration wave in the following year.

unique applications. An outside package may allow a fast start to the change process and avoid unnecessary confusion and lost time, but never covers all the bases. The partnership between the consultant and the hospital requires mutual effort in order to bring about the synergistic creativity present in the best applications.

Implement Recommendations for Organizational Renewal

The implementation wave allows executives to power up business performance. The program provides a creative destruction process that removes old philosophies, policies, and practices, and gives birth to a new, more powerful culture. The program inserts a new and dynamic problem-solving approach that starts with managers and is then cascaded through all levels of the organization. The targets are improved Customer service, increased morale, smoother operations, faster innovation, and better financial performance.

As managers gain skills and begin to alter the organizational culture, they turn their activities toward changing work systems and fixing Customers' needs and Associates' grievances. The solution of these problems in turn leads to a flowering of the culture, strengthening both managerial skills and resolve.

Creating and Implementing Solutions

As recommendations for change come in, barriers to approval and implementation must be dealt with. Under this model, nearly all recommendations are funneled through the MAC (see Figure 11.2). The expectation is that nearly all DIG recommendations will be approved. In the early rounds, before people have gained experience with the technique, some recommendations are sent back for rework but this problem tends to fade in time.

Recommendations generated by DIGs are authorized at two different levels. If the recommendation involves several departments that have agreed to it, and if it does not require additional dollars or people, then the MAC has authority to

Figure 11.2. DIG System Work Flow.

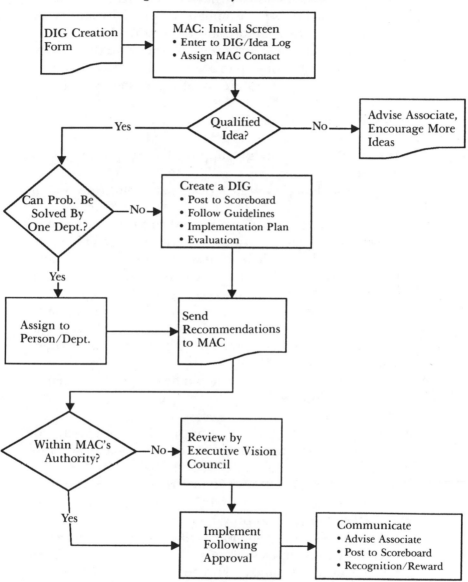

Source: S. Sherman and K. Weidner, *Guidelines for Do It Groups* (Inverness, Ill.: Management House, 1991), p. 41.

approve the recommendation. If, however, the recommendation requires additional dollars or human resources, or affects the total organization, then authorization is required by the Executive Vision Council. Some organizations authorize the MAC to approve recommendations up to a specified dollar amount.

The following criteria are usually considered in the review process, and idea submitters are asked to check how well their project measures up:

- Any change must fit or support the corporate values statement.
- Procedural changes must be designed to improve one or more KRAs.
- Changes in one department should not cause a negative impact in another department or with outside affiliations unless these changes have been dealt with in the proposal.
- The proposal should return more than the salary cost of the people making the change—ask, Is it worth doing?
- Opportunity costs are weighted heavily in prioritization.
- The proposal must fit organizational goals, or at least not be at variance if it has emerged "out-of-time" with other planned changes.
- New procedures or policies should be designed to enhance overall operating efficiency.

Other economic factors affecting approval are availability of funds, whether the item was budgeted or unbudgeted, how rapidly the project will recover its cost, and what the opportunity-cost picture looks like. Projects that strongly favor Customer satisfaction or quality, or that would be beneficial to Associates, stand a better chance for approval.

Approvals are time-bound, with the MAC required to make its decision within a week. Any decision that has to go to the Executive Vision Council is limited to two weeks. Some New American Hospitals have even built in fun penalties of $5 assessed against each member of the Executive Vision Council for being unable to reach a decision on a recommendation within the time period! Others give the MAC decision authority if the

Vision group doesn't act in time! The point of making change is to make change! At first the pace seems dizzying, but it soon becomes the norm. Approval rates in recent applications of the model run around 90 to 95 percent.

Keeping Change Cooking with MAC

The roles, tasks, and procedures of the various in-house coordination groups have been discussed earlier. As recommendations from managers begin to pour in, usually at a rate of a few hundred each month, and as the DIGs begin their work, it's important to grab hold of this mushrooming wave of change. At first the participants are full of an unorganized energy and the program runs on raw excitement. But unless this is coordinated soon, there is a risk of losing the heady start out of the gate.

The MAC speedily gathers project recommendations, sets priorities, and starts DIGs or makes individual assignments. Deadlines are set: it is helpful to check on how things are going. More important than the project work they are doing is the need for all participants to have a success experience—a win. This is essential, for it teaches that they can attack a problem and prevail.

Keeping Change Talking with CAC

The CAC speedily communicates the onset, the process, and each new result of the change initiative. In this case, communication is aiming for commitment, not just information flow. An intensive internal public relations campaign is aimed at all Associates, and a real battle for the hearts and minds of the people must be waged. One of the best ways to build political support is to trumpet the successful gains being made. Publish every win, every positive step. Convince everyone within the corporate family that the right direction is being pursued.

Successful campaigns have featured weekly newsletters, daily Change-Grams on cafeteria tables, unit Communication Centers, Stand and Deliver meetings where the president makes decisions on-the-spot to those with change needs, and videotaped presentations about the change that are broadcast over in-house TV.

The most successful efforts have taken place when the communication stream is unrelenting. The intensity of this effort is necessary both to shift deeply ingrained attitudes and perceptions and to adequately cover the torrent of change.

Keeping Change Smiling with SAC

The SAC speedily moves to establish a series of socialization events that break down inhibitions and barriers. Later on, the emphasis will be on celebration of results, but at the beginning the task is to make people comfortable enough to work together. Initially the SAC focuses on managers' needs as they go through management development together. But as the change wagon starts rolling, the SAC soon finds itself sponsoring celebrations of DIGs and individual achievements. By expanding its focus to cover Associates, it helps to socialize and network supporters of change.

The SAC does not replace the social activities function for the hospital. Instead it focuses on the people who are involved with organizational change. By reserving its activities only to contributors, it creates a new "in group." Opportunities to play hard are designed for those who work hard. Another function of the SAC is to help maintain morale during the change period. Change tends to create anxiety, and celebration is a solid way to reassure people that things are going to be just fine.

Producing Results Quickly

Because of the uncertainty surrounding major organizational change, it's imperative to get points on the scoreboard early. Find things that can be done quickly. Look in particular for something symbolic, a sore thumb that's been irritating a large number of people. Your political supporters do not need another study or a promise that somehow things will begin happening in mañana land (a common failure of many TQM programs). They need to see something soon. Quick results give program supporters belief in the process that's being undertaken.

Of the many ideas recommended in this book, which might be most helpful in meeting this need? What worries the managers most? What are doctors most upset about? What makes Associates unhappy? From this list, pick some that are small enough to be doable — balance importance against feasibility, and be wise enough to know that very large, complicated problems should not be addressed at the program's onset when skills and culture are weakest.

As resistant groups or individuals are encountered, if there is an issue important to them to which you can lend your support, you may be able to quiet their resistance on other aspects of the change program. You must give a little to get a little. Every manager should be instructed to find such issues early in the change effort in order to increase buy-in.

Off with the Old, On with the New

Zapping hated policies, irritating practices, and old-fashioned ways of doing things accomplishes several goals. First, it removes a misfitting element from the organization and lightens the load. Second, it affirms to program supporters that the change effort is serious and emboldens them to go and do more. (One president gave out cap pistols with notches on the handle when a manager accomplished five kills.) Finally, it signals to those resisting change that it's going to be increasingly difficult to live in the old culture. By destroying the time clock, burning the policy manual, or doing away with privileged parking spots, it's possible to communicate far more effectively that the old day is over.

It's equally important to communicate using symbols of the new culture. When DIGs become widespread, their presence is a message that your thinking is respected. Many positive messages come into being that are received as symbols of the New American Hospital. Awards, true celebrations of achievement, more ennobling job titles — all signify the new day.

Picking Targets Carefully

In the beginning of change, managers pick targets of opportunity, things that they want to fix. As Associates join the process,
they, too, go after their own agendas. Since these are intelligent
and trustworthy folks, this nearly always works to the advantage
of the organization. However, to some extent it also means that
the change projects are not completely under the direction of
the organization.

To provide balance to this free-form surge in creativity, it's
important to look at the list of needs that those responsible for
the program initially drew up in the preparation wave. Just
reading this book will produce a list of hundreds of specific
changes that could be considered for implementation. In addition, leaders will want to insert their ideas. To discover these
other needs, the MAC posts its own DIG topics and makes
individual project improvements. If this is not done, the management machine is not built and the culture is inadequately
altered to support change later on. In addition to this free-form
target shooting, add in the structure that provides overall balance to the process.

Key Issues for the Executive Vision Council

The Executive Vision Council becomes an important element in
implementation since it is responsible for program oversight
and for handling some of the tougher problems and key issues.
Experience suggests that the following issues may arise.

The Problem Manager. It's not unusual for a small percentage of the management staff in any organization to refuse to
move with the organizational flow to the new culture. Management of problem performance remains with the chain of command, not the MAC. If bottlenecks in performance routinely
occur with the same individuals, a plan to correct this performance should be created. If performance continues to fail, the
manager will need to be removed.

Inappropriate Financial Control. It's not possible to fund
all the changes people want to make. The successful financial

executive will balance the need to show budget restraint with idea groups by finding a way to redeploy assets within the budget, suggesting ways to implement pieces of the project, and, at all costs, avoiding unthinkingly turning down innovation by automatically saying, "We can't afford it."

DIGs Used as Dumping Grounds. Sometimes individuals or departments form DIGs as a way to heap blame on another department, or, more commonly, they dump problems into a DIG that ought to be solved within the department. A DIG is not a substitute for correct management of the department. When Executive Vision sees this, it needs to point out to all concerned that this is old hospital thinking.

The Runaway MAC. The MAC is not a new layer of management. Its power stems from its advisory role to the executives, and from the interpersonal and persuasive skills of the members. On rare occasions, the MAC can begin to overly advocate change in a way that creates a control problem for executives. This usually happens because of poor selection of members who did not understand the need for good political functioning. What is called for is clear coaching, clear expectations, and the formation of a true team interaction between the executives and the MAC. The risk is small and usually preventable.

Cascading Organizational Change

Initially the focus is on developing the management group, but development of the organization calls for the involvement and commitment of all levels. There are several ways in which all other parties can be tied into the overall change effort. A general sequence would be to bring the following groups into the effort as follows:

1. First-line supervisors
2. Associates and volunteers
3. Physicians and the board
4. Customers

Cascading Prescriptions for Supervisors

This is the true working level of management. Enlisting these people solidly in the change agenda is critical. Many organizations simply include them with managers in the management development sessions, blurring any distinctions between the groups. The following ideas are ways to include supervisors:

- A complete or abbreviated management development program for first-line supervisors is necessary to get them in sync with the rest of the management team.
- Political forums and processes must be established to give supervisors greater sway in both departmental and interdepartmental problem solving. Restructure management meetings to include their voice.
- Completion of training modules on adherence to values and their application, DIGs, and new role authorities is needed.
- New rating and reward systems must be explained, to understand what pays off in the New American Hospital.

Cascading Prescriptions for Associates and Volunteers

Experience has shown that there are similar needs for both Associates and volunteers. As volunteers become increasingly involved in hospitals that need their contribution, they have become a second work force. Associates and volunteers react positively to:

- Programming that outlines what the New American Hospital is all about, its major philosophies, and how the changes will both affect and involve them.
- Completion of training modules on values adherence and application, DIGs, and new role authorities.
- Explanation of new rating-and-reward systems — what pays off in the New American Hospital. This does not apply to volunteers.

- Plans to involve Associates in DIGs with managers early in the program. This should be done on a wide-scale basis and should involve 75 percent of the staff by the end of the first year. Participation is the best route to buy-in. Volunteers may participate as they are able.

Cascading Prescriptions for Physicians and the Board

Some physicians and board members will participate in DIGs and may even offer to chair a DIG. Wider participation on DIGs by physicians is usually *earned* by the organization as it improves functioning and servicing of medical staff concerns. Medical staff leaders and board members are frequently invited by executives to sit in at management training sessions; the common experience is that a few members will attend and spread the word to their colleagues. Some of the severest critics and skeptics of the change effort have become its greatest champions. Helpful actions include:

- Programming that outlines what the New American Hospital is all about, its major philosophies, and how the changes will both affect and involve them
- Completion of training modules on adherence to values and their application, and inclusion in DIG training for those who are interested

Cascading Prescriptions for Customers

Customers can be very helpful in creating a change wave in the organization. They are most helpful as a change force at the point in the process where managers and Associates are beginning to run out of ideas and energy. The presence of Customers in the organization's functioning helps to get everyone back on target. Meetings of the Committee of Excellence become a major social opportunity in which friendships and relationships are built between people who heretofore may have interacted with the hospital only on an individual Customer-receiving basis. Helpful actions include:

- Programming that outlines what the New American Hospital is all about, its major philosophy points, and how the changes will both affect and involve them. The media approach and message content are differentiated from those given to staff. Brochures, in-house patient education, waiting-area videos, and news releases all carry the new message.
- Establishment of Customer Committees of Excellence or Customer Councils. These can be used either as focus groups or advisory panels.
- For those who are interested in becoming involved in problem-solving groups, completion of training modules on values adherence and application, and inclusion in DIG training.

Baseline and Outcome Measurement

Change measurement is important to ensure that the renewal effort is achieving its objectives as well as to show members of the organization that they have achieved considerable success. Beyond these purposes, it is important to demonstrate the financial returns and other values of the initiative. Finally, measurement identifies what has not been accomplished; this is valuable knowledge to have in figuring out what to do in the next wave of organizational change.

Recording Gains on the Cafeteria Scoreboard

The Victory Scoreboard approach is an excellent means of tracking progress in the organization. The CAC designs and installs the Victory Scoreboard no later than the beginning of Module 2. The scoreboard should be very large, perhaps the length of one of the main walls within or outside of the cafeteria. There are four recommended categories on the scoreboard:

1. DIGs to Do
2. DIGs in Progress
3. DIGs Done and Approved
4. DIGs Implemented

The DIGs to Do category lists the unsolved problems. Generally, these DIGs are still looking for membership or chairs. Once the DIG membership is complete, the Scoreboard indicator moves to the DIGs in Progress category. When the DIG has returned its recommendations to the MAC, the indicator is moved to the DIGs Done and Approved column. This indicates only that the analysis and recommendations are complete. When recommendations are fully implemented, the indicator moves to the DIGs Implemented category. This simple method lets everybody know what's going on and visually demonstrates both that change is occurring and that the total amount of change is immense. Everyone visits the board to see the progress of their favorite project or to take in a hoopla celebration when a DIG is implemented.

Identifying KRA Measures

It is valuable to monitor key management and organizational performance during the transformation. If you can show positive movement in terms of Customer satisfaction ratings, productivity numbers, financial performance, and innovation rates, you are demonstrating the effectiveness of the renewal effort.

The old American hospital relied on financial measures to judge the organization's vitality. These measures are valuable, but they are too gross to measure many of profitability's antecedents. There is a lag time between what we do to improve Customer satisfaction and our later ability to capture it as a correlated impact on financial performance. The New American Hospital needs more effective measures to better predict where future financial performance will be going. New American Hospitals set up a matrix of measures for each of the seven KRAs that track progress toward preset goals. (See Exhibit 2.1.)

In one hospital, a relatively simple, broad-based measurement of Customer satisfaction showed that at the onset of organizational renewal, Customer satisfaction ratings were in the 70 percent range. This measure jumped over 20 percent on average across the departments measured. It was not unreasonable to predict that this organization's financial performance would also improve as Customers passed along the news that this organization had greatly improved in its ability to satisfy Customer needs.

Instituting Performance Measurement

The key point of measurement is to create an orientation toward results that focuses both people and work priorities. The New American Hospital is often less interested in being sophisticated than it is in being effective. If your choice is to use a fairly simple system that can be up and running now as opposed to some perfect system that may be available in the year 2015, go with the simple system now.

Identifying what outcomes are wanted starts people thinking about what they can do to affect those targets. Once they know what the boss is going to be looking at, it's amazing how people fine-tune their radar to point in that direction. Focus people on the results you want by measuring KRA outcomes and feeding this information back to the troops. Measurement changes behavior markedly when there are consequences at your end and good people at the other end.

The touchdown can only be celebrated when people know that the goal line has been crossed. Make sure that there are some early measures of the key things that need to change in the organization. When the changes happen, we can break out the champagne and have a party. If they don't happen, we'll know that our efforts have been unfruitful so far and we must try something new.

Feedback to management is less important than feedback to Associates. Post performance measures in the unit, and, where possible, make a chart or a graph of them, rather than columns of numbers. Use this instrument as a powerful communication tool. Keep it short, keep it simple, and keep it relevant. Let Associates and managers use it as their tool. Too often in the old hospital, information was kept in the hands of a few. Executives played the "confidential" game and kept information from their people. Information in the hands of a few executives is not as valuable as widespread dissemination of useful information in the hands of the many.

Once the measurement system is up and running, refine it. Managers who were initially asked for their input into the creation of the measuring system should now be allowed to make refinements as the change progresses. If additional numbers are to be recorded, program the computer to monitor them. Run some simple correlational statistics to find out if you have too many measures that are in fact measuring the same thing. Measures tend to start crude, rapidly grow in complexity and variety, and then fall back to a few key statistics that prove to be the most useful over time.

Calculating Return on Investment

A number of TQM, guest relations, and other programs have been undertaken with noble purposes, but little in the way of documented return on investment. It's important to recognize that we do not improve the organization just because it's fun, or even because it fits our values; it's done to make a substantial difference in business results. Unless it gets those results, the intervention is a failure.

The renewal program adds value to an organization's business interests by producing a number of changes that improve internal business efficiency and external market impact. Clients' experience is that cost savings in the way of system improvements begin almost immediately, build through the program, and continue for some time afterward. *If it is done right, the program will return more than its cost within the first year.*

The change program outlined here affects a wide range of variables in the organization's culture, operating systems, leadership style, structure, and staff utilization. Unlike academic research, which concerns itself with the results of changing a few variables, this planned intervention affects literally hundreds of variables within the organization. Compounding the difficulty of being able to demonstrate that these variables are producing a return is the fact that there are a number of intervening variables, factors in the organization between the input of the change variables, which management largely controls, and the resultant outcomes the organization desires. This is the real world of management, a world where reasonable assumptions are used to make changes in a planned way in order to achieve desired results, but where this has to be done in a complex organizational setting with many pressures and complications.

Field experience shows that program returns are real. It's best to recognize that some results are "hard" and some "soft" in terms of measurability. While the question of proof is difficult, results can be demonstrated and measured if the client is willing to track a number of key indicators.

Hard Measures of Return on Investment. Where possible, establish baseline measures prior to the program's onset. The easiest way is to use existing monthly or quarterly statistics that are already part of the information system, supplementing them with special tracking efforts. Don't expect measures to show an immediate response. Some will begin to change soon, some will change by the end of the program, and some will continue to change after the program ends. A minimum two-year measuring effort is suggested, measured from just before onset.

Existing productivity measures can be used to measure changes over time. However, older productivity measures may be inadequate to assess the dynamics of organizational change. For example, true registered nurse productivity would increase if they were allowed to focus on patient tasks alone, but if errand-running staff are added, the FTE count might not drop. To say that measurement may be problematic is not to beg the question of whether productivity is improving. Productivity will increase as a result of renewal, but the complexity of the equation may call existing measures into question. What can be measured?

1. *Increased Customer satisfaction.* Customer satisfaction indexes should be taken no later than three months into the

changeover. Client experience has shown large rating gains as the system of patient care is debugged and staff attitudes improve.

2. *Market share.* Calculated by major market segment, market share should increase as a result of a better organization, all other factors in the competitive arena being constant. Improvements in organizational excellence may be offset by better marketing or technology by the competition. This key statistic should begin to shift about one year into the change.

3. *Increased financial performance.* Measures of gross revenue, expenses, and net margin may or may not show improvement because of decisions made in the organization and the market, so it may be better to look at submeasures such as waste reduction and unit productivity. The gross financial statistics are easily available, however, and ought to be part of the measurement package. Changes will not occur immediately but there should be some, assuming that other factors affecting organizational performance remain somewhat steady.

4. *Reduction in operating costs.* An audit of operational cost-containment elements is conducted by all managers as part of the change model. To determine savings, a dollar value is usually estimated by a panel of managers. The volume of ideas and changes will number in the hundreds to thousands, so the expected value will be substantial. Cost containment will be both direct and indirect in savings impact.

5. *Elimination of nonproductive meetings.* An early project is to identity all meetings, their costs, and the results obtained. This project will usually net savings approaching $1 million in medium-sized organizations.

6. *Increased productivity and quality levels.* While the change program is not entirely a productivity management or quality control system, Customer satisfaction standards of performance are increased, worker participation in Customer Satisfaction Teams and on DIGs is greatly enhanced, and productivity enhancements and quality improvement

methodologies are actively worked on throughout the program.

7. *Decreased number of lawsuits.* Legal and disciplinary actions should be fewer, accompanied by a lower dollar value for the average legal action.

8. *Improvement in morale.* The creation of a superior working environment for all Associates leads to a number of positive effects on business. Dwight D. Eisenhower said, "In war, the most important weapon is morale." Opinion survey information as baseline data prior to onset is ideal, with postmeasurement showing expected double-digit percentage gains in the average category response for both Associates and managers.

9. *Turnover rates.* Turnover should decrease as the work climate improves. This means less cost for recruitment, training, and overtime in units during vacancies as well as higher morale among work teams that function without losing key members.

10. *Length of employment before turnover.* This is a secondary measure of turnover impact.

11. *Employee vacancy rates.* Recruitment draw from the labor market should increase as the climate improves. Part of recruitment savings is represented in "ease of recruitment," as well as in decreased overtime and use of outside agency staff.

12. *Elimination of problem Associates.* A housecleaning opportunity exists in the program for retooling or removing problem Associates. A standard formula is used to calculate the cost of current problem Associates.[2] First, survey managers for the total number of problem Associates in their immediate chain of command, and, of these, the number that should be terminated. Calculate these numbers as a percentage of the total work force, and multiply by 8. Multiply these eightfold percentage factors against the total Associate payroll to see the total dollar drag on the organization. For example, if problem Associates represent 5 percent of the work force, and the organization has an annual payroll of $10 million, the total damage to the organization represents approximately $4 million.

13. *Increased number of suggestions.* Ideation statistics are typically not monitored by old hospitals, so it may be difficult to establish a baseline. As these measures are established, a healthy increase in their rate of growth should be seen. Ideation represents future Customer and Associate satisfaction, and business success.

14. *First-year value of DIGs.* Several hundred DIGs operate during the length of the program. An attempt should be made to estimate only their first-year value. Discount the total savings by the percentage of the problems that would have been solved without renewal. If the estimate is that 20 percent of the problems would have been solved anyway, discount the estimate by 20 percent.

Soft Measures of Return on Investment. There are other expected areas of financial return and other nonfinancial benefits. These are sometimes measurable but often subjective in determining the degree of change accomplished or placing a value on the changes achieved. One approach to measurement would be to list the following items and then survey managers about the degree of improvement or dollar worth represented by the changes. *If you could go out and buy these items for your organization, what would they be worth to you?*

1. *Greater managerial and departmental productivity.* Creation of a common management system: Managers and units accomplish more results with a management system than without it. This can be tracked by the quantity of projects completed by quarter, as well as by the number of DIG completions.

2. *Narrowing the range of leadership style.* By better defining good management practice, there is a reduction of leadership dissonance and less performance slippage. This leads to greater team cohesiveness, communication, and relaxed interaction.

3. *A "can do" atmosphere.* When the attitudes and motivational levels of the managers are fired up, the group becomes more energetic and independent.

4. *More on-target thinking.* Creating superordinate goals for the causes of organizational excellence, Customer service, and

team respect means being sidetracked less, requiring less supervision, and having fewer false starts.

5. *Increased physician recruitment capability.* The quality of the staff and morale are often cited by physicians as the primary reasons they choose a particular hospital in which to practice. This is subjective on the part of the recruiter, but it is borne out in the percentage of job offer acceptances and positive responses to invitations to practice.

The aggregate value of these hard and soft indicators will prove or suggest a correlation to the program's intervention that cannot be ignored. Clients' estimates of return on investment vary, depending on how many measures are tracked, but they are between five and twenty times the program investment cost for value received in the first twelve months. For example, an in-house study of managers at St. Mary's Medical Center in Evansville, Indiana, showed an aggregate estimate of $5,724,390 in the intangible benefits area.[3] This included the use of a common management system, better communication, clearer goals, and improved motivation. This first-year result in a large hospital was about ten times program cost. This soft finding correlated with hard indicators that showed an increase in Customer satisfaction from 62 percent to 77 percent during the same period in terms of those describing service as "excellent," a drop in Customer complaints of 50 percent, and a 2 percent market share gain. In addition, there was an increase of $19.2 million in net patient service revenue and a $2.4 million increase in excess revenue over expenses. Other indicators showed little or no change or were not measurable at the time. Management's conclusion was that the renewal effort was worthwhile, even though its measurement was not entirely accurate or possible.

Notes

1. K. von Clausewitz, *On War* (Bergenfield, N.J.: Penguin U.S.A., 1968).

2. C. Sherman, *From Losers to Winners* (New York: AMACOM, 1988, pp. 15–16).

3. *Return on Investment Study* (Evansville, Ind.: St. Mary's Medical Center in-house study, 1992, p. 31). The study compiled the estimated value of intangibles in terms of the renewal program's impact and measured as many other hard measures as could be obtained.

12

Accelerating the Change Process

Faster. Higher. Stronger.
— Olympic motto

The normal response pattern in organizations at the conclusion of implementation is to want to take a pause. The perception is that the job is done and it's time for a rest. However, the only thing finished is the initial training; the organizational change process is still under way. How to carry on becomes the key problem. Table 12.1 shows the phases of the acceleration wave — the outline of this chapter's contents.

Retargeting

Retargeting becomes the starting point for staying on-track. A one-day planning conference should be held at the conclusion

Table 12.1. Acceleration Wave.

Phase	*Objective*
Retargeting	Drive business results
Institutionalizing change in systems and culture	Solidify organization development gains
Unleashing the power of customers and innovation	Improve organizational responsiveness
Intensifying systems improvement	Improve decision making, speed
Deepening management and Associate development	Build on management strengths
Driving change with evaluation and rewards	Better focus performance
Revisiting structural design	Improve accountability

of the implementation wave. The Executive Vision Council and selected other participants go through a detailed agenda to determine wins and losses.

Critiquing the Implementation Wave

Exhibit 12.1 shows the coverage of one such meeting. At this point measurement data are helpful to see differences in organizational performance before and after implementation. Return-on-investment information is also useful in energizing the critique panel to take on more change.

The primary focus of the retargeting session is looking forward. The major output of the conference is a new work list and a change management plan to carry it out. For retargeting to be effective, several objectives need to be accomplished:

- Identify what items of work and areas of emphasis need to be addressed in the next year.
- Examine the adequacy of the new systems; ask what's working and what isn't.
- Identify change supporters and devise ways to reward them and celebrate their accomplishments.
- Identify change resisters. The time for patience is at an end and key personnel decisions must be made.
- Clearly understand what change failures occurred, and redirect the change effort.

Common Implementation Problems

During critique sessions a number of problems emerge that are typical for organizations doing renewal work — usually they only amount to a few in any given change effort. Some of these problems might have been controllable. Others were either uncontrollable or idiosyncratic to the particular institution. Would you anticipate any of these in your organization?

Exhibit 12.1. Excerpts from a Retargeting Conference Agenda.

---

1. Critique summary
   What did we achieve? What's different with managers, Associates, Customers, the organization?
2. Have we built a field of dreams, or of weeds?
   What is the unfinished work agenda?
   Are we still committed to excellence? Is change under way?
   7-S retargeted needs (strategy, systems, staff, style/symbols, structure, shared values, skills)
   Do we need to accelerate change in year two?
   What are our dreams for getting to the twenty-first century?
3. The lean, mean management machine: Are we fully functioning?
   How do we need to work better as a team?
   Is it time to replace managers or executives?
   Are we ready for advanced system-improvement techniques?
   DIGs and the idea engine: Is innovation alive?
4. Arnold Schwarzenegger management
   Using development to strategically build the business
   Executive individual development plans (IDPs) and advanced management program for year two
   What change forces need enhancing? What new goals are needed?
5. Oakbuilder options for cascading
   Avoiding the risks of a stalled organization development effort
   Have we won the hearts and minds of Associates? Physicians?
   What communication and education pieces are needed?
   Associate development to achieve full operational impact
   Accountability: Measurement-and-reward systems
6. Customer as king
   Where have we not completed Customer retrofit of our system?
   The Customer as change master: Customer committees and Customer satisfaction teams
   Strategic Customer response: Who owns the problem?
7. Rethinking the effectiveness of macro systems
   Does the strategic-marketing plan drive change?
   Are budgeting, financial efforts, and MIS helping managers?
   Is the organizational chart helping get work done?
   Is Human Resources improving the work force's capabilities?
   Building on Beliefs: The Motorola example
8. Future roles
   MAC, SAC, CAC—justify the group's existence and present goals
   Executive role: MBWA, cheerleading, finding the right work level
   Are managers running free, or do barriers need removal?
   What new organization development change and renewal mechanisms do we need?

- Uneven attention is given to different KRAs; some need more emphasis.
- Too many projects are in process; not enough are finished to provide a sense of pride in performance.
- Certain vice presidents' areas are lagging behind the rest of the organization. There is lack of program support in one or more segments of the hospital.
- Inadequate executive attention is being paid to the non-operations work of strategic planning, marketing, and finance. The organization still struggles because it isn't any better as a business, even though it has become better internally as a system.
- There is division between the MAC and the executives, usually caused by a nonassertive MAC or by executives who are resentful of having their decisions challenged. They show immaturity as people, amateurity as leaders.
- Human Resources is swamped by the amount of work required in that area; needed pieces are not completed in a timely manner.
- Problem employees linger. While this problem was addressed early in the program, it is taking too long to get rid of them due to slow processing or managers shy from the task.
- There is inadequate follow-up by some CEOs and vice presidents. Lack of structure at the top breeds carelessness down the line.
- Executives are not turning over adequate budget authority, pushing approvals lower, or releasing information.
- The CEO is too slow in replacing managers or making structural changes. The usual reason is a vague hope that somehow things will improve. They don't.
- As part of the Customer service strategy, executives are assigned the discontinuance of dog services. Failure to do so continues to create organizational drag.
- There is difficulty finding people to serve as DIG chairs. This problem is often traceable to a lack of payoff for the chairperson; it becomes an unrewarded duty.

Why Change Programs Fail

Research shows that many organizational change programs fail due to their complexity. While New American Hospitals efforts have succeeded at a 97 percent rate, it has often been the case that one or more of the following elements has given us fits. Common failure points suggest *areas of vulnerability*, things to watch out for:

1. *Lack of executive leadership*
    *   Inadequate dissatisfaction (*D* in the change formula) on the part of executives and lack of long-term commitment. Halfhearted, they start programs but fail to carry through.
    *   Failure to remove or manage problem executives and managers in a timely way. Their power is in their passive resistance to the change; they are insulators who deaden the flow of change energy through the organization's circuits.
    *   Lack of follow-up enforcement on new directions, decisions, procedural changes, and behaviors. Organizational drift ensues.
    *   Misuse of the change opportunity, defense of the status quo, or a tendency to sit on the sidelines like a spectator rather than participating. This is a consistent pattern with a minority of vice presidents.
2. *Poor managerial performance*
    *   Insistence on maintaining old enmities between departments and key players. This residue of old battles often poisons the well of attempts to build team play. These managers fail to understand, "That was then; this is now."
    *   Adopting a "this, too, shall pass" mentality; waiting out the program. Too many "program-of-the-month" experiences in the past sometimes cause an immunity to further change.
    *   Inadequate socialization and celebration; maintaining old-hospital glumness. The new model tells people to

work hard and play hard, but some find job joy hard to come by.

- Lack of consistent discipline in living the new behaviors. Occasional performance leads to spotty results.
- Feeling that workers, not management, are the problem. In hospitals this is often expressed by blaming an in-house union or difficult doctors. Managers project blame rather than owning the problem.
- Failing to make the renewal effort a part of normal business activity. Saying, "It's not my job." This failure is shared with the executive level.

3. *Inadequate performance by consultants or change agents*
- Underestimating the enormity and complexity of carrying out a major change program in the middle of running an ongoing business.
- Underestimating the client's need for a cookbook approach. Organizations need more turnkey pieces than they or the consultant initially thinks.
- Underestimating the need for manager and chain-of-command "workarounds" to get at the truth. Relying on the chain of command alone to make change happen is a disaster.

4. *Poor business environment*
- Finding that area competitors are simply too good or fast in bringing new products to market. They swamp the organization in the midst of its renewal effort.
- Being caught in a financial squeeze, unable to provide the seed money that innovation requires. Cost containment becomes so severe that it squeezes the life out of the organization.

None of these factors are unmanageable, but they require work and time. Part of retargeting is figuring out how to deal with these issues. If the implementation wave had some of these difficulties, now is the time to address them as the organization prepares to enter the acceleration wave.

Institutionalizing Change

The positive changes achieved must be "locked in," as well as the means that produced them. At the same time, you do not want to replace the old rigidity with a new rigidity. How can you ensure that the self-renewing managing that has been inserted into the organization will remain? In too many instances, a new CEO enters an organization only to reverse the direction taken by an earlier leader. Is it possible to attain a "government of law, not of men"? The answer is to institutionalize change so that positive management does not become subject to whim.

Systems and Policy Formalizes

By changing organizational systems, job descriptions, and roles and putting everyone in small groups, a widespread change in understanding takes place that affects how people think. This can be formally cemented through such channels as replacing policies, changing the technology people are tied to, and setting up new decision-making rules. Ask yourself: How could we cement this change in place and make this way of doing things the norm people have to adhere to?

Policy is not welcome in the New American Hospital if it is restrictive and a substitute for brains. But policies that require adherence to values, support Associate ideation and participation, and mandate systems can be helpful. These policies are supported in turn by Associates and Customers; popular policy — the right kind of organizational law — is hard to overturn.

Education Cements

"An educated citizenry is the best defense against tyranny," wrote John Adams. The New American Hospital sells its ideas to the organization through indoctrination and education. Its story has to be told anew to each entering member of the staff, and its living reality has to pay off on the job.

Explain New American Hospital philosophy and values during the selection process, intensively beat the drum in orientation, and make continuing education a sacred cause. Create forums for open discussion, amplify the messages coming from the in-house press, and create human growth through wide-scale development. When people buy the concepts and are intelligent and informed, the culture becomes almost impossible to overturn.

A classic case occurred when a board mistakenly hired a CEO who talked New American Hospital lingo but who wasn't of that persuasion. Within a few months he was undoing many of the gains that managers and Associates had worked so hard to forge. In another time they might have just acquiesced, but once they had tasted freedom it was a different story.

The phones began to ring off the hook at board members' homes. Petitions were circulated among Associates requesting the man's removal. Members of the medical staff joined in, vowing to publicly revolt if changes that had benefited them were allowed to regress. The board chairman later recounted that the only uprising he'd ever seen that could approach it was when Alexander Dubček was overthrown in Czechoslovakia! The hapless CEO was gone in four months!

The Power of Customers and Innovation

While much work is done on Customer problems during implementation, directed by the values and KRA concepts, there is a need to intensify the Customer focus and the innovation that feeds it in the acceleration wave.

Forming Customer Satisfaction Teams

One successful approach is the creation of a Customer Satisfaction Team (CST) in each department whose size and mission make it feasible. Management delegates the most important KRA to a team of Associates and empowers it to do what's needed. The group might suggest the formation of new DIGs, make individual assignments, start training programs, or survey Customers. It does not implement projects as much as it manages the KRA. Some describe it as a departmental MAC. Others note that it places management responsibility in the hands of Associates. The department manager retains approval authority over recommendations but usually serves to advise and to approve resources. (For a full description, see Chapter Four.)

In one particularly difficult implementation, the CEO became unhappy with a very resistant management team. For complicated reasons, half of the entire team eventually had to be replaced. Because they were so uncooperative, the president decided to set up CSTs in the first year instead of the second, but he went beyond just Customer issues. He called them KRA teams and told managers that groups of Associates would now make all decisions in the unit including those relating to budget expenditures! As amazed supervisors looked on, the teams took over and, with little stumbling, did a very adequate job. As the president said later, "In getting the job done, just do what ya gotta' do!"

Taking responsibility for virtually the complete running of the department is the concept of semiautonomous work teams. It is a goal that is reachable if the culture permits and encourages it, if information and educational support are available, and if group members have become experienced in small-group processes. A CST is a more limited and less risky approach; it is valuable in getting organizational response to the Customer because the organization is under the direct control of those who provide the service. Watching your staff function at such a level becomes one of the finest moments in your management career.

Raising Customer Satisfaction Standards

If the Customer Satisfaction Index standard of 95 percent set in the first year is now being attained, and it often can be, then raise it. How high? Ask the group. Squeezing out the next two or three percentage points is often as hard as covering the distance from 85 percent to 95 percent. Departments have to put a fine edge on an already good effort and then dig deeper to eradicate more subtle faults in the system. Every percentage point gained at this level deserves a gala celebration!

Starting the Idea Engine

A suggestion system that permits Customer input is usually not initiated until manager and Associate recommendations have been pursued. When that cleanup is done, the idea engine is begun (see Chapter Five). In our conceptualization, this usually falls near the end of the implementation wave, around twelve months into the program. The idea engine is a major idea-gathering mechanism open to all staff, Customers, visitors, and physicians. Our judgment is that to begin this system earlier would be a mistake because of the backlog of problems that staff need to pursue, and because the DIG system is not yet fully developed. By focusing on DIG development first, you allow the problem-solving groups to become fully functional by the time the Customers unleash another tidal wave of suggestions.

Multiplying Processing Groups

This acceleration dynamic is critical: the objective is to obtain widespread involvement by Associates and to sustain the change momentum. Our experience in helping executives lead change is that momentum lost is not easily rebuilt; continuous accelera-tion of change is the best way to build the new, highly par-ticipative organizational culture.

To keep momentum up, increase the number of groups of all kinds (DIGs, Customer Councils, new management groups, and task forces). Also increase the speed of decisions and finesse in implementation so that people see good results as soon as possible. At the same time, don't overreach or skate so close to the edge that control is lost. I'm often asked how many DIGs an organization can run *at any given time*. The range seems to be around seventy-five in organizations with a thousand Associates. Some people are between group assignments, and there's always the press of other work. The actual number your organization can accommodate has to be found experientially. Raise the number until the strain begins to show. Settling for fewer DIGs retards progress.

In the acceleration wave, increase total problem-solving

activity in both quantitative and qualitative terms. That doesn't mean just having groups for their own sake. Examine the percentage of total Associates who served on at least one DIG. If the first-year goal was 75 percent, raise it to 90 percent during acceleration. (Experience suggests that 100 percent is not attainable, since a number of Associates do not want this kind of involvement.) Another way to raise the bar is to increase the average number of problem-solving groups served on by each Associate. Again, the pursuit of numbers is not as important as the quality of the results, but it is a measure that invariably accompanies true acceleration. This is also the time to look at how well groups are functioning. What additional training is needed? What additional tools, skills, and capabilities do they require?

Intensifying Systems Improvement

Near the end of the implementation wave, the organization should be introduced to new approaches that refine existing operations. These tools and techniques include:

- KRA CI (continuous-improvement methods)
- Work Simplification (basic industrial engineering principles)
- Managing Small-Group Dynamics (advanced DIG management)
- Problem Solving and Decision Making (specification and matrices)
- Refinement of the evolving measurement system

Experience has shown that these tools are not supported or used well until cultural change has taken place (see Chapter Five). We've also learned that many problems the hospital initially faces don't need advanced or deeper methods in order to solve them—there are many commonsense, simple things that need to be cleaned up. In fact, these sophisticated acceleration wave techniques actually serve to retard the speed and quality of change if they are used during the implementation wave!

During implementation, groups focus on smaller and more doable problems. Advanced problem-solving techniques are usually not required to address these garden-variety problems. Empowerment plus common sense is often all that's needed to hammer out a solution. These problems are the "apples on the ground, close to the tree" that Deming speaks of. Letting groups solve them quickly gives confidence to the participants and credibility to the process. It also avoids the problem of a too-slow start to the change process that has most often accompanied traditional TQM approaches. Fixing the obvious doesn't require a ponderous system or an overreliance on an unnecessary systems approach. However, as the cleanup proceeds, it uncovers harder and harder problems that often require more powerful tools. It is at this point, either near the end of implementation or at the beginning of acceleration, that quality-improvement processes should begin.

Deepening and Intensifying People Growth

Under the changes made in the first year, there has been an increase in skill and confidence. Now is the time to extend those gains.

Revisiting Management Development

Management development is not an acute need in the second year, because it was heavily covered during implementation. Our usual recommendation is to allow between four and six days of additional seminar programming. What's needed are topics that extend the range offered in implementation and add to critical managerial skill development, such as:

- Personal and Managerial Productivity
- Sizzling Selection and Realistic Retention
- Managerial Problem Solving and Decision Making
- Managing Stress, Strain, and Dis-Ease
- Developing Human Assets and Potentials
- Cost Containment and Systems Improvement

- Managing Creativity and Innovation
- Planning and Control of Operations
- Managerial Communication and Negotiation
- Time Managing for Results

This is also the time to make hard decisions about team makeup. People who have not performed should now be removed from supervision. There may be a place for them doing technical work, or perhaps it will be time for them to move on. If they didn't conform to the new culture's requirements after a year of development, they won't conform to it later.

Associate Development

The bottom 50 percent of the work force is where an organization wins. Associate development becomes more intensive in the acceleration wave. Topics to be inserted into the organization include those needed to support the change process (DIG operations, value-centered managing), courses on tools and techniques to support technical specialties, and courses in continuous improvement.

As outside change agents, we work hard with top management to gain support for in-house education. Usually, a telling argument can be made for education having high return on investment and for the idea that a highly educated work force will present fewer control problems. We suggest train-the-trainer workshops on a range of skills and knowledge that will raise organizational capabilities.

Increase the training budget, in terms of both dollars and hours of training per Associate. As decision making moves downward, the educational support required increases. This financial and time cost is always returned by way of increased work and quality output. What did you spend last year? Budget a minimum of 100 percent more this year. Make whoever is responsible for this activity measure the effectiveness of the programs so that not one thin dime is spent on mush. The total training effort must be directly related to the work at hand, not on off-task programming. Provide a larger budget, but demand more results.

Driving Change with Evaluation and Rewards

In the first year, much of the change is carried just by enthusiasm and the novelty of newly gained empowerment. These will remain the prime drivers in the acceleration wave, but more formal approaches to the evaluation of people and results, and reward systems that can pinpoint specific performance needs, can function like a second-stage rocket booster. I disagree with those who try to drive organizational change just by tinkering with rewards and incentive plans. More structure and additional systems are needed, making the rewards-only approach insufficient for adequate change. But I strongly agree that modifying the reward system can be a powerful driver. (See Chapter Thirteen for a full discussion.)

The beginning of the acceleration wave is the ideal time to start making substantial changes to the reward system. Generally, it seems to work well to add in the elements I have discussed earlier in this book a piece at a time in an evolutionary approach. As new pieces are added, there is a novelty, a feeling of new fun things we can do to win payoffs. None of these programs should take away from the feeling that all payoffs are geared toward solid work accomplishment—that is, they should support the prime emphasis on attaining excellence and not be allowed to be seen as trivial or unconnected from solid work.

Revisiting Structural Design

Early organizational design issues were first discussed in the preparation wave. If no action was taken to alter existing reporting relationships then, now is the time to revisit the question. The objective is to collapse levels and consolidate departments to obtain faster workthroughs. If that was accomplished at the outset or has partially evolved during implementation, all that may be required now is some polishing. (See Chapter Seven.) Now is definitely the time to look again at the temporary coordi-

nating groups that were put in place to help get the organizational renewal effort accomplished—the MAC, SAC, and CAC.

Reconstituting the MAC

Restructuring of the MAC, or at least some rotation of membership, is needed by the beginning of acceleration. This rotation allows managers to get back to departments that have been
struggling in their absence. It also brings new ideas and perspectives onto the MAC. Rotation may be indicated if members have
used up their political I.O.U.'s, have not been as effective as was
hoped, or have been promoted to vice president. The latter
situation happens often—high visibility plus an effective performance equals promotion!

The MAC may need to be restructured because of a
change in the mission. At the beginning, when the organization
was just entering renewal, a great deal of early coordination and
education needed to be done, DIG startup was at hand, and a lot
of confusion existed. Now, a year later, the MAC is faced with
different challenges. DIG volume has become overwhelming,
managers are feeling fatigued, and the problems that need to be
solved are more difficult. Because the challenges are different,
talents needed on the MAC may also be different. The MAC
might also bring on first-line supervisors or Associates as members, another sign of cascading representation.

Because of the volume of change occurring at this time,
some MACs reform into KRA Councils. A KRA Council is a
smaller group of three to five managers and Associates who
focus on a single KRA. All DIG requests, suggestions, and complaints relating to a KRA are directed to that group. Depending
on the hospital's size and the volume of change needed, there
might be as many as seven KRA Councils, or there might be
three or four with each group handling more than one KRA.
The KRA Council chairpersons are usually members of the
MAC, which functions as an overall coordinator and direction
finder.

While the MAC was originally conceived as a temporary
coordinating structure, executives usually decide to keep it

going after the original changeover. The MACs value, in the many different forms that have evolved, has been sufficiently great so that organizational leaders have asked them to continue — a vindication of the hypothesis that a greater managerial voice in hospital operations has long been needed.

Revitalizing the SAC and the CAC

Ideas for what to do with these groups other than membership rotation are less clear. The duties of the CAC have sometimes been folded back into the areas of marketing and public relations and education. When that occurs, the new communication channels and media tend to be maintained as part of an enriched product offering; there is a greater use of newsletters, closed-circuit TV, and Associate orientation programming. More often, the CAC continues to function through the acceleration wave as a separate entity. This judgment is made by executives according to what works best.

SAC functioning in this period tends to follow an expansion mode. Sons of SAC spin off, or multiple SAC groups arise. Socialization is so powerfully effective with managers during the first year that it makes obvious sense to use it as a change tactic with Associates, as cascading covers larger and larger groups of people. SAC groups tend to be organized to serve either target populations, such as nurses, or special interests, such as sports leagues. A key point to remember is that the primary purpose of the SAC was to assist change, not just to run recreation programs or do fun things. The SAC must remain focused on helping the organization's renewal effort.

13

Driving Change
with Rewards

> No man who continues to add something to the material,
> intellectual and moral well-being of the place in which he
> lives is left long without proper reward.
> —Booker T. Washington

Putting in place the massive change that is the New American
Hospital is no small task. In order to change how the organization performs, it is first necessary to modify and shape how
people behave. One of the powerful forces that must be elimi-
nated is the pattern of old hospital pay practices, which conditioned people to act in ways that were not good for them or the
organization. It is also useful to rethink how evaluations are
used to affect behavior, and who should do them. Last, new
reward schemes need to be added to challenge and add zest to
living and working in the organization.

Modifying and Shaping Behavior

Based on E. L. Thorndike's work, one can articulate two laws of
human behavior that can significantly support efforts to change
the organization:

> 1. *Behavior that is reinforced is likely to repeat.* That
> means any behavior, good, bad, or indifferent. If
> hospitals pay people for "being sick," or reward
> them for time away from work, then absenteeism
> will flourish. The probability of this prediction
> happening is very strong.

276

2. *Behavior that is not reinforced is likely to extinguish.*
That also means any behavior, good, bad, or indif-
ferent. The term *extinguish* here is used to mean to
go away or die off. The probability of this predic-
tion is less strong. Nurses not recognized for their
contributions may continue to do good work because they are reinforced by their own sense of
professionalism, but many simply leave nursing
feeling unappreciated.

The basics of behavior modification are contained in these two
statements. As a manager or executive trying to make change
happen, you must add as much reinforcement as possible
around the new behaviors that are desired. What behavior do
you want? What reinforcement will you provide if you get it?

It's also important to remove any reinforcement for wrong
behaviors or for behavior that is counter to what is desired in the
New American Hospital. What behavior should disappear?
What is supporting that behavior now, and how can that reinforcement be removed?

Managing the Three R's

The three R's of management are *recognition, reinforcement,* and
reward. Just as education has its fundamental three R's, in the
area of motivation, the three R's are essential and vital to redirect
and cement appropriate behaviors in place. In this book the
terms are often used interchangeably, but there are certain
distinctions. *Recognition* is usually a visible, audible signaling to
somebody else that a certain behavior or achievement has been
noted. It feeds the ego of the other person and adds to her sense
of self-importance. *Reinforcement* is anything that lets the person
know he's on-track with some behavior. Brief comments such as
"That's right" or "Very good" are reinforcing. *Reward* is usually
the act of giving something tangible, such as a bonus for a
special performance or achievement.

In most hospitals, three-R management is very poor, and
what is rewarded is often inappropriate behavior. Because there

is little money available, it's important to get the most impact possible. To drive home the changes required in the New American Hospital changeover, it will be important to systematically clean up errors in the human reward picture and to add extensively to the pattern of reinforcement.

Instituting a Three-R System

A supervisory three-R system is made up of several elements. First, an MBO approach is taken that matches work assignments to a subsequent reward. Exhibit 13.1 illustrates an approach to releasing motivation that assigns growth-stretching work, holds the supervisor accountable for providing elements of support such as training, and then targets a reward for the successful completion of the assigned project.

Second, a list of rewards is created that are in the supervisor's control to administer. Most of these are no-cost or low-cost items; they should be primarily nonfinancial in nature. We work with client organizations to develop a list of approximately three hundred recognitions and reinforcements that might be given, a list that can be quickly referenced as the occasion demands. Some recognitions are fairly standard, but they range all the way up to more creative and wacky ideas:

Three R's for Associate Performance
- Valet parking by manager
- Being allowed to spend time in another department
- Newspaper ad telling of appreciation
- Lunch served by manager
- Letter of appreciation to the Associate's mother
- Lawn mowed by manager
- First choice on vacation schedule
- Dedication song on the radio
- Permission to attend or chair board meeting
- Star on name tag
- Special parking space
- Flowers sent to spouse
- Shoes shined by manager

Exhibit 13.1. Managing Motivational Release.

Managing Motivation Release
MANSYS℠ The Integrated Management System

Manager _____

Unit _____ Date _____

Associate	A. Individual Motivation Planning		B. Manager's Response Planning		C. Group Dynamics and Team Focus
	Key Talents/Strengths to Build On	Significant Assignment, Authority Upgrade, or Achievement Opportunity	Obstacle Removal or Special Support Needs	Reward, Recognition, Reinforcement Contingency	
					1. The team that works together grows together. What task force approaches can be taken with work at hand?
					2. Feedback changes behavior. What nonthreatening measures of group performance will be provided?
					3. They need you. What coaching, group training, or mentorship will you provide?
					4. MBWA: What obstacles need to be cleared to permit more time with the troops?
					5. What's a heaven for? What group reward or ceremonies are due?
					6. Job joy: What are the socialization opportunities this quarter?

Source: Management House, Inverness, Ill. ©MCMLXXXV Beta Group, Ltd.

- Role of department manager for the day
- Chocolate kisses
- Office door or work station decorated
- Free physical, or other hospital service
- Barrel of popcorn
- Roving plaque or trophy
- Free hair styling
- Free oil change
- Free round of golf, bowling pass, movie tickets
- An evening of baby sitting
- Gift from the gift shop
- Free cafeteria meal
- Decorated cake announcing the achievement
- Billboard ad (this is cost-effective for multiple thank-you's)
- Night on the town

A budget is established for these items, and those that cost a little more are reserved for more significant accomplishments. Local merchants are often willing to donate free chits for merchandise.

The third element is to train supervisors to give three-R feedback at the rate of eight times per day for an average-sized unit. We've selected that number based on a number of studies that show that high-producing supervisors do this eight times per day, whereas low-producing supervisors typically issue reinforcement once per day. The concept here is to set an expectation that the stream of communication coming from supervisory personnel is one that appreciates, rather than depreciates, the value of humans at work. Once this element takes hold, the palpable feel of departmental communication is notably improved.

Finally, each supervisor in the three-R program sponsors social events in the department. While this is less motivating than individual recognition, it provides a supportive human ambiance that adds to the pleasure of doing great work. It is wonderful to work in the New American Hospital where creativity and work are celebrated, and where efforts to grow enhance personal worth.

Stopping Old Pay Practices

The inappropriate use of financial payments must be stopped so that scarce resources can be better used to shape and modify behavior in the direction required by the rapidly changing organization.

Stop COLAs, Step Increases, and Useless Payments

Immediately stop all cost-of-living adjustments (COLAs) or step increases. These payments for nonperformance came out of old personnel administration models whose aim was to keep salary grades current with existing labor market conditions. It was easy administratively to move all registered nurses up ten cents an hour after three months. This administrative convenience, however, costs great amounts of money and indiscriminately rewards both good and bad performers. The good performers wind up thinking: Why am I making exactly the same money as Jackie, who does half the work that I do? Why, when I volunteer for extra shifts, don't I get any more money than the others? How can a person who is a problem in this organization be granted a cost-of-living increase? These comments and questions cannot be answered. Remember the rule: feed your friends, not your foes. Some people not only don't deserve more; they deserve less!

One way to decrease people's pay is to not give them a merit increase. With normal cost-of-living escalation, a person's pay actually decreases over time. If some Associates are worth less in their performance than others, shouldn't their pay provide less compensation? By doing away with COLAs and step increases, all dollars available go into the merit pot, or into bonus payments used to reward desired behaviors. If we took all the salary dollars that these outdated systems pay to marginal Associates, the total is often more than enough to fund many of the bonus payments we'd like to make to the real winners!

The marginal performer who receives a COLA has been rewarded and reinforced for these marginal behaviors! This intensifies and solidifies poor performance. Since we would prefer to rehabilitate Associates rather than terminating them, if we really want to get their attention, it's best to withhold rewards as a preparation to getting them back on-track.

Give Increases and Bonuses for Merit Alone

While it is implicit in the discussion on stopping pay for nonperformance, the organization also needs to implement and educate Associates on the concept that no money is paid except for meritorious performance. Cash payments must be directly linked to desired performance on the daily job or in particular need areas or points of emphasis that executives consider worthy of application, and for no other purpose. Some hospitals have longevity bonuses. While this is a matter of judgment, my opinion is that no one should be paid a longevity bonus. The fact that people have been employed for a long time may simply be a reflection that they couldn't get a job anywhere else and no one had the guts to fire them. Recognize seniority, and give long-term Associates honor and all due respect, maybe even a trip to a resort, but actual cash should be reserved solely for meritorious performance.

Slow Down Evaluations, but Stay Competitive

Without announcing a freeze on jobs, a de facto slowing down of the organization's promotion and evaluation processes could be helpful during organizational renewal. The organization has to learn that the basis on which a person is promoted and the behaviors that pay off are different. Stop promoting people simply because they've been there longer or are the best technical workers. Slow down changes in employment status that are based on evaluations that came out of the old system. Holding these processes up gives the organization a little time to think through how it wants to evaluate people and what it wants to promote them to do.

It's not possible to wait too long. The organization has to stay competitive with the opportunities that are available in competing organizations. Holding back on merit increases and other rewards as the organization begins its transition sends a very powerful message. Identifying what the boss will pay for now becomes the topic of conversation in the informal world.

Driving Behavioral Change
with New Evaluation Approaches

Feedback changes behavior, but changing who provides the evaluation feedback, and then tying it to rewards, *really* changes behavior! How can evaluation procedures and criteria be changed to help the process of growing people and the organization?

Performance Self-Review

People who do a job forty hours a week are eyewitnesses to their own performance; supervisors see a substantially smaller sample of the total work performance. It is important for Associates to think through the question: How well am I doing on the important tasks that must be done? The New American Hospital makes Associates responsible for thinking through how well they're doing and making suggestions for improvement in their performance. Whatever performance review system is currently used in the hospital should be converted to a self-review in which Associates fill out the performance evaluation form and bring it to their supervisor for review and counsel.

The supervisor retains the authority to change any ratings he or she does not agree with, but this is seldom necessary. The vast majority of Associates rate themselves at about the same level the supervisor would or lower. This is another example proving that if Associates are treated like adults, they become thoughtful evaluators rather than passive recipients of the "grade."

Performance evaluation systems have to be changed to include the values as the first section on the form. If Associates aren't meeting the values, what difference does it make how well they're technically doing their job? Job performance aspects are rated second. Many of these technical performance indicators can be grouped under one or more of the KRAs, and some New

American Hospitals have included a KRA format as a way of spelling out the job in accordance with restructured job descriptions, which also often follow this same format.

Deciding Who Determines Pay

Behavior follows rewards. Merit pay systems attempt to tie pay to performance, but the impact varies depending on who does the evaluating. When the supervisor is the evaluator, the employee's behavior has to be focused on pleasing the boss. Some supervisors may penalize the person who fails to cozy up to them or who has different ideas and is willing to fight for the good of the cause. On the other hand, the manager often finds that while people may be working hard they sometimes lose sight of primary objectives such as serving the Customer, or they may be insensitive to key relationships like working with other team members.

One modification of a pay-for-performance system would be to include some rating of the Associate by Customers or teammates. If the Associate's performance is rated by Customers so that half of his or her merit pay is determined by Customer ratings, the result is an incredible sensitivity and desire to satisfy Customers' demands! Or if some substantial percentage of pay is determined by ratings from fellow workers, the Associate learns, and learns immediately, to become supportive of the team.

Under any of these approaches the role of the manager is to act as a checkpoint in case the group dynamics go sour. I recommend that managers use this pay scheme on an experimental basis. The evidence suggests that groups are very effective at monitoring their own behavior and at regulating and appropriately allocating resources to the members of the group who deserve it. These ideas, like so many in the New American Hospital, are both sensible and experimental. Don't be afraid of trying the new.

Using Customer Ratings to Determine Merit Pay

One idea worthy of note is to use Customer ratings, either individual or departmental, as a partial determinant of merit pay or profit-sharing bonuses received by everybody within that unit. If a department's internal or external Customers rate it at 98 percent favorability, doesn't it deserve a greater merit allocation or bonus award than a department that is rated at 79 percent? This concept grants executives much more forceful control over managerial and departmental ratings than almost any other system I've seen.

For example, assume that two departments, A and B, have the same total amount for salaries and the budget allows for a 5 percent total merit pay increase. If department A received a 98 percent favorability rating from its Customers, 98 percent of the merit allocation money would be granted to the department. However, the department that received the 72 percent favorability rating would have its merit pay reduced 28 percent. In this way, the organization is saying, "When your Customers are happy, I'm happy to reward you. When your Customers aren't happy, expect to pay for it." This tends to make the group dynamics operate in one of two ways: teams will pull together or they will turn on the individual performers or supervisors who are causing the problem. In either event, the executive is in a winning position to either assist team formation or bring to a head the need to clean house.

Executive Pay: Quality, Customer, and Associate Ratings

Since behavior follows rewards, it becomes particularly important to consider the basis on which executives are paid. Historically, boards have looked at financial performance as the primary criterion — if the organization is making money, things can't be too bad. The reality is that short-term gains or this year's fancy accounting footwork can mask a host of problems and organizational dry rot. Suppose that executive pay is determined by ratings of existing quality, Customer satisfaction, and Associate morale. High quality and happy Customers are proof that the organization is producing the kind of results that will eventually lead to increased market share and higher sales. Associate ratings, on the other hand, quickly spot poor leadership. The remaining portion of executive pay can still be based on financial performance.

What is sometimes needed is to shake executives out of a too narrow focus. If their pay is heavily determined by how well Customers are satisfied, you can bet that they will be out of the office a lot making sure the Customers are satisfied. Executives will also build some very strong measures of Customer, Associate, and quality outcomes in the organization so that they can quickly spot errors and omissions. When the executives are only evaluated on their financial performance, to some degree they can ignore Customer service, treat Associates badly, and damage the organization in other ways.

Allowing Associate Ratings to Affect Executives' Pay

When reward-and-evaluation processes cascade downward in the organization, it is possible to radically alter first-line supervisors' behavior by having their merit pay or bonus amounts determined by ratings from their Associates. When the ratings affect a sizable percentage of a supervisor's pay or bonus, it tremendously changes his or her behavior toward Associates. The fear that supervisors will simply try to run a popularity show has not been borne out in my experience.

Customer ratings of a supervisor can also be included as a source of merit determination, leading to increased urgency in Customer response. When an entire management team knows that it will be reward starved unless it alters all existing policies, procedures, and practices that get in the way of Customers or Associates, it becomes a hit squad, energized to blow up barriers. This encourages managers to do the work they want to do to revitalize our hospitals.

Adding New Reward Schemes

Too many hospitals depend too much on the merit pay system as the primary way of rewarding people in the organization. A whole host of new reward schemes, primarily nonfinancial, should be added to build new and needed behaviors. What might they include?

Rewarding Heroes for Living Their Values

As a change strategy, it's essential to center the organization around its values. To obtain that behavior, create awards for each of the values and for the total values statement. One hospital created awards for each of their values (STEP: Service, Team, Excellence, People), along with an overall award for the department that best reflected STEP in its entirety. Rewards were given monthly within departments, and quarterly housewide. Awards were generally nonfinancial, such as plaques or other items left in the department where others could see them. The purpose of the awards was not only to recognize individual performance, but to teach others what would be rewarded in the future.

By themselves, values remain only an intellectual concept until they are brought into reality through dedicated examples. By telling stories about those who have been heroic in the struggle, executives can show the living examples that are the lifeblood of cultural change.

In addition to orientation, signage, and reward programs, it's important to incorporate values into the organization's human resource systems. Make a rating of the values the first section of the employee performance appraisal form and the first section of the pay increase or promotion recommendation form. Tie the values into the warnings given to problem employees. In nearly all cases, problem employee behaviors are violations of one value or another and should be given preeminence in terms of the importance of the offense. If the values of service, respect, or excellence are considered to be the corporate religion, violating them is worse than breaking a policy; management systems ought to reflect this.

Giving Awards for KRA Work Objectives

KRAs are the work the organization is trying to accomplish. While this is initially a management concept, KRAs are everyone's responsibility. The experience in New American Hospitals is that Associates quickly memorize the KRAs and help tremendously in curtailing work drift; every Associate functions like a manager. If people become recognized for results in the KRAs, the work force learns that results, not activity, are what we have to focus on. Awards can be issued for each of the seven KRAs. When respect, recognition, and rewards are tied to achieving significant results there is a double win: the person who succeeds is recognized, and the organization gets the benefit of the Associate's accomplishment.

In the New American Hospital, managers use a work plan in which quarterly work objectives are spelled out. Those who achieve objectives on a timely basis should be rewarded better than those who continually fall behind their deadlines or don't achieve adequately. An annual merit review makes rewards too distant, a year away from what the manager may be doing today. On the other hand, if the manager knows that a certain list of tasks must be accomplished within the next ninety days, and that some quarterly bonus or evaluation point is available, he or she continually pushes for results. Just changing the schedule of how rewards are earned quickens the pace of organizational change. Most executives whom I have worked with want a lot of change and want it now. To facilitate this it's necessary to quicken the reward schedule.

Giving budget freedom to achievers is also a powerful reward for managers. One hospital allowed managers who met KRAs, such as 95 percent Customer-satisfaction ratings, to be exempt from budget cuts. Another spin was to create a variable quarterly budget funded by 5 percent reductions in budget from managers who did not meet enough of their quarterly objectives.

The old hospital often demonstrated the listlessness and lack of aggressiveness toward the task that typifies reward-starved cultures. In the New American Hospital, executives and department managers are always looking for a way to use the three R's in the completion of any significant project. Rewards might include a dinner, a party, or an executive visit to the department — anything that massages the ego and lets people know their work is appreciated. Rewards must not only happen once in a while. Managers should always be thinking, "If the work gets done, here's how I'm going to reward the people who did that work." Show people that it's worthwhile to undertake new assignments, rather than having them feel like a gladiator who's had to fight the lions ten times in a day with no applause.

Providing Payoffs for Attendance, Education, and Suggestions

Special reward or recognition schemes can be targeted to behaviors that are of strategic importance to the organization. Rather than paying people for being sick and absent from the job, and thereby reinforcing them to stay home, why not pay them starting on the second day of their sickness? This covers the person who is truly ill and follows the insurance company concept of not paying for first-dollar coverage. The money that is saved by not paying for the first day is then paid out in bonuses to people who attended 100 percent of the time, thus creating an incentive to be at work. The lost-time patterns in American hospitals are horrendous compared to those of other industries. The reward system is the reason: the time abuser gets all the money and the person who is there all the time is not rewarded.

To motivate Associates to further their careers, upgrade their skills, and gain the education they need for a rapidly changing future, New American Hospitals add an educational bonus; this is a slight adjustment in base pay or a one-time bonus payment after completing a set number of hours of continuing education. Some organizations go even further and require a set number of continuing education hours in order to be eligible for a merit pay increase. Yet others require merit pay increases to be tied to a demonstration of mastery of new information or skills.

A third area that might be driven to greater levels by manipulation of the reward system is the suggestion rate. Since we need a lot of suggestions and people to work on the small groups that spin out of that input, the system should include a range of recognitions that is based on the number of suggestions given, the value of those suggestions, or the category into which a suggestion falls. Points accumulate with each suggestion, and additional points are added if the person making the suggestion works on a problem-solving group, or if the suggestion is implemented. Reward each behavioral step in the suggestion process. Smart management knows that you can do a lot of work by setting up systematic reward systems and making work fun.

Promoting Only from Within

Promotion represents the biggest reward a person can receive for meritorious performance. If selection processes have been good and qualified people are found in abundance in the organization, there should be a large enough personnel pool in all but the smallest departments to allow promotion of staff people into supervisory positions. When people are not promoted, a deadening of motivation is created in the person who has worked hard hoping to get ahead in the organization, and it creates additional morale death through organizational stagnation — people staying too long in jobs in which they've gone stale.

One clearly sees this in hiring young M.H.A.'s to fill top spots; this sends a loud message to all department heads that they are in a dead end job. Over the decades this practice has frustrated many department heads who have learned that they cannot move up. The argument that department heads aren't ready for hospital executive positions is specious. Nobody is ever ready for a new job. No one is initially qualified to be president of the United States. Life is learning. The effective organization is one that prepares people and narrows their developmental gaps. Identifying the people with potential for being promoted, providing on-the-job stretching assignments, encouraging additional schooling, and pushing the growth button hard quickly creates a ready tier of replacements. As people move upward and experience the fruits of their labor, they bring an enthusiasm, fresh approaches, and liveliness into the organization.

Adding Nonfinancial Rewards

New American Hospitals have recognized people for accomplishments such as the greatest number of ideas submitted, the largest number of Customer thank-you notes received, or perfect attendance. There are Daring Greatness trophies, Lady with the Ax awards (based on a story from the life of Florence Nightingale), and membership in the President's Academy. How about an award for the most improved department, the highest number of training hours per Associate, or Best Innovation of the Year? Pick the behaviors you would like to see in the hospital, then work backward to build a nonfinancial reward system that features them.

While these nonfinancial rewards and honors may have some cost (tickets to the ball game, an educational seminar, a weekend resort trip), actual cash payments should be saved for result-getting behaviors only. Teach the lesson that the only way to increase pay, be promoted, or in other ways be rewarded for behaviors is to do the job or some aspect of the job extremely well. Don't give out money for just being there another year, or because somebody down the hall got a raise.

Making It Fun with Socialization and Celebration

McDonald's has a vice president of fun, IBM a vice president of socialization. These are plum assignments, and a lot of us would like to have them! As part of their reward system, Apple Computer took all five thousand of its Cupertino, California, home office Associates to see the movie *E.T.* These organizations understand that if we play together, we stay together, and that to work hard, we have to play hard. Have you been allowed to play lately? All work and no play is a good way to describe failing hospitals. The organization that can shake out the wrinkles and stand back from the intensity of its labors, laugh, and enjoy itself is going to win against all competitors. I'm not talking about the ho-hum annual picnic or the jaded Christmas party, but about creativity in play and the celebration of achievement.

One way to think of socialization is as another kind of work. The organization that does this work, and does it well, makes all the other work infinitely easier. Socialization builds friendships, ventilates the organization, and lightens the load. Laughter is the best medicine for many of the difficulties the hospital industry is experiencing. There has been too much gloom, too much fear, and too much anxiety, and it is paralyzing people. This has created an oppressive climate. An organization that does not do the fun work is an organization where all the other work is infinitely harder to achieve.

A particularly important form of socialization is celebration of particularly significant achievements, of individual, departmental, or organizational objectives that have been attained. We need such celebrations; they are sustainers of our corporate society. The New American Hospital practices KISMIF — Keep It Simple, Make It Fun. Making it fun is the great sweetener that adds levity and joy to accomplishment.

Some New American Hospitals have done such zany things as have a skyjumper drift earthward to present a Captain Marvel sweatshirt for an achievement — SHAZAM!!! Another brought in a fortuneteller to promise good fortunes to those who met objectives, lived values, and responded to other messages worked into her fortune-telling spiel. Still another had "Credo Man," complete with red suit and cape, lead cheers from different sections of the management team as they recited their values and toss out lightning bolts to note good deeds. Another organization interrupted its management meeting to have Superman come in complete with soundtrack and lighting effects to reward super performances. The zanier and more creative these events are, the better. We ought to have fun and enjoy ourselves; it's part of life and ought to be part of our job life. But we are also canny enough to know that it is good management. Points made in jest are often the most powerful — such moments are teaching moments.

Regularly Rotating and Refreshing Rewards

Individual, departmental, and organizational rewards should be rotated on some periodic basis. Effective organizations try variations of old programs or use a program only for a period of time and then substitute something new. People like to play Monopoly, but they don't like to play it every day of their life. If they can still pass Go and collect the $200 by playing in a chess tournament or mastering poker, they will do it. Variety is the spice of life, and the reward system needs to show variety if it is to continue to have impact. It's not uncommon for executive councils to put monitoring of the organization's reward system on their agenda for monthly review; they play with the reward system all the time. It's a real spur, one of the most potent tools to effect change in a significant way.

Ask, What behavior do I want? What performance do I want? How can I reward that behavior so that I can get it? This is the habitual mindset of the successful executive. Create new reward categories at every turn. There's nothing that says these things have to have eternal life. Make it fun. "You may have already won $10,000,000," is the kind of message that sure makes me open my envelope!

When I started to write this book I knew there had to be an end. Let me finish where the change effort must begin, with hospital leaders and great Associates facing a difficult job.

Leadership in the New American Hospital requires a vision that will serve to challenge and unify the organization's people for the assault on Mount Olympus. In its simplest terms, people working in every hospital want to spend themselves in a meaningful quest for excellence, to give themselves to work that matters so that their very lives will matter. In the New American Hospital, people sense that they are on a road that is going somewhere, and that the effort is worthwhile. While the problems of health care are unclear, what is clear is that we can do things a lot better than we are now and that many are willing to take the risk. The hidden army of change agents waits for the leaders who will call them to the battle. For our Associates, for the Customers we serve, for our own sense of worthiness, for our children, and for America, it is a time for greatness.

Recommended Readings

The following reading list has been organized to correspond with the chapters of this book because these sources have particularly important messages related to the content of *Creating the New American Hospital*. While the readings listed below have other important information, they are helpful as springboard material for this book.

1. Why Hospitals Fail

Coile, R. C., Jr. *The New Hospital*. Rockville, Md.: Aspen, 1985.
de Bono, E. *Tactics*. Boston: Little, Brown, 1984.
Goldsmith, J. C. *Can Hospitals Survive?* Homewood, Ill.: Dow Jones–Irwin, 1981.
Porter, M. E. *Competitive Advantage*. New York: Free Press, 1985.
Steiner, G. A. *Strategic Planning*. New York: Free Press, 1979.
Toffler, A. *Power Shift*. New York: Bantam Books, 1990.
Toffler, A. *The Third Wave*. New York: Bantam Books, 1990.

2. Reinventing the American Hospital

Bennis, W., and Nanus, B. *Leaders*. New York: HarperCollins, 1985.
Cox, A. *Straight Talk for Monday Morning*. New York: Wiley, 1990.
Crosby, P. B. *The Eternally Successful Organization*. New York: Plume, 1988.
Deal, T. E., and Kennedy, A. A. *Corporate Cultures*. Reading, Mass.: Addison-Wesley, 1982.
Gardner, J. W. *Self-Renewal*. New York: HarperCollins, 1963.

Harmon, F. G., and Jacobs, G. *The Vital Difference*. New York: AMACOM, 1985.

Hickman, C. R., and Silva, M. A. *Creating Excellence*. New York: Plume, 1984.

Kiam, V. *Going for It!* New York: Signet, 1986.

Leebov, W., and Scott, G. *Health Care Managers in Transition: Shifting Roles and Changing Organizations*. San Francisco: Jossey-Bass, 1990.

O'Toole, J. *Vanguard Management*. New York: Berkley, 1985.

Peters, T. J., and Waterman, R. H. *In Search of Excellence*. New York: HarperCollins, 1983.

Shortell, S. M., Morrison, E. M., and Friedman, B. *Strategic Choices for America's Hospitals: Managing Change in Turbulent Times*. San Francisco: Jossey-Bass, 1990.

3. Unleashing People for Contribution

Fear, R. A., and Chiron, R. J. *The Evaluation Interview*. (4th ed.) New York: McGraw-Hill, 1990.

Hersey, P. *The Situational Leader*. New York: Warner Books, 1984.

Kingsley, D. T. *How to Fire an Employee*. New York: Facts On File, 1984.

Kirkpatrick, D. L. *How to Improve Performance Through Appraisal and Coaching*. New York: AMACOM, 1982.

Lawler III, E. E. *High-Involvement Management: Participative Strategies for Improving Organizational Performance*. San Francisco: Jossey-Bass, 1986.

McGregor, D. *The Human Side of Enterprise*. New York: McGraw-Hill, 1960.

Sargent, A. G. *The Androgynous Manager*. New York: AMACOM, 1983.

Sherman, V. C. *From Losers to Winners*. New York: AMACOM, 1987.

4. Delivering the Service Strategy

Albrecht, K. *Service Within*. Homewood, Ill.: Dow Jones–Irwin, 1990.

Blumberg, D. F. *Managing Service as a Strategic Profit Center.* New York: McGraw-Hill, 1991.

Carlzon, J. *Moments of Truth.* New York: Ballinger, 1987.

Davidow, W. H., and Uttal, B. *Total Customer Service.* New York: HarperCollins, 1989.

Glen, P. *It's Not My Department.* New York: William Morrow, 1990.

Liswood, L. A. *Serving Them Right.* New York: HarperCollins, 1990.

Peters, T., and Austin, A. *A Passion for Excellence.* New York: Random House, 1985.

5. The Quality-Productivity-Innovation Equation

Blake, R. R., and Mouton, J. S. *Productivity.* New York: AMACOM, 1981.

Geneen, H. *Managing.* New York: Avon Books, 1984.

Grove, A. S. *High Output Management.* New York: Vintage, 1985.

Guaspari, J. *I Know It When I See It.* New York: AMACOM, 1985.

Harrington, H. J. *The Improvement Process.* New York: McGraw-Hill, 1987.

Ryan, K. D., and Oestreich, D. K. *Driving Fear Out of the Workplace: How to Overcome the Invisible Barriers to Quality, Productivity, and Innovation.* San Francisco: Jossey-Bass, 1991.

Walton, M. *The Deming Management Method.* New York: Perigee, 1986.

6. A Streamlined Management System

Batten, J. D. *Tough-Minded Management.* (3rd ed.) New York: AMACOM, 1978.

Beck, A. C., and Hillmar, E. D. *Positive Management Practices: Bringing Out the Best in Organizations and People.* San Francisco: Jossey-Bass, 1986.

Douglass, M. E., and Douglass, D. N. *Manage Your Time, Manage Your Work, Manage Yourself.* New York: AMACOM, 1980.

Drucker, P. F. *Managing for Results.* New York: HarperCollins, 1964.

Drucker, P. F. *The Effective Executive*. New York: HarperCollins, 1966.

Jenks, J. M., and Kelly, J. M. *Don't Do, Delegate*. New York: Ballantine, 1985.

LeBoeuf, M. *Working Smart*. New York: Warner Books, 1979.

Mackenzie, A. *The Time Trap*. (rev. ed.) New York: AMACOM, 1990.

Perry, L. T. *Offensive Strategy*. New York: Harper Business, 1990.

Schoenberg, R. J. *The Art of Being Boss*. New York: HarperCollins, 1978.

Seiwert, L. J. *Time Is Money: Save It*. Homewood, Ill.: Dow Jones–Irwin, 1989.

Silber, M. B., and Sherman, V. C. *Managerial Performance and Promotability*. Inverness, Ill.: Management House, 1984.

Sloma, R. S. *No-Nonsense Management*. New York: Bantam Books, 1981.

Sloma, R. S. *No-Nonsense Planning*. New York: Free Press, 1984.

Winston, S. *The Organized Executive*. New York: Warner Books, 1983.

Winston, S. *Getting Organized*. (rev. ed.) New York: Warner Books, 1991.

7. Optimizing Organizational Structure

Adizes, I. *Corporate Lifecycles*. Englewood Cliffs, N.J.: Prentice-Hall, 1988.

Ouchi, W. G. *Theory Z*. Reading, Mass.: Addison-Wesley, 1981.

8. Leading the Transition

Adair, J. *Effective Leadership*. Aldershot, England: Gower, 1989.

Belasco, J. A. *Teaching the Elephant to Dance*. New York: Crown, 1990.

Bennis, W. *On Becoming a Leader*. Reading, Mass.: Addison-Wesley, 1989.

Cribbin, J. J. *Leadership*. New York: AMACOM, 1981.

Gabarro, J. J. *The Dynamics of Taking Charge*. Boston: Harvard Business School Press, 1987.

Gabarro, J. J. *The Dynamics of Taking Charge.* Boston: Harvard Business School Press, 1987.

Harris, P. R. *Management in Transition: Transforming Managerial Practices and Organizational Strategies for a New Work Culture.* San Francisco: Jossey-Bass, 1985.

Koestenbaum, P. *Leadership: The Inner Side of Greatness.* San Francisco: Jossey-Bass, 1991.

9. Managing Wide-Scale Change and Reconstruction

Alberti, R. E., and Emmons, M. I. *Your Perfect Right.* (6th rev. ed.) San Luis Obispo, Calif.: Impact Publishers, 1990.

Beer, M., Eisenstat, R. A., and Spector, B. *The Critical Path to Corporate Renewal.* Boston: Harvard Business School Press, 1990.

Brown, A., and Weiner, E. *Supermanaging.* New York: McGraw-Hill, 1976.

Cohen, H. *You Can Negotiate Anything.* New York: Bantam Books, 1980.

Fisher, R., and Ury, W. *Getting to Yes.* New York: Penguin, 1983.

Grover, R. *The Disney Touch.* Homewood, Ill.: BusinessOne Irwin, 1991.

Iacocca, L. *Iacocca.* New York: Bantam Books, 1984.

Kanter, R. M. *The Change Masters.* New York: Simon & Schuster, 1983.

Kimberly, J. R., and Quinn, R. E. *Managing Organizational Transitions.* Homewood, Ill.: Irwin, 1984.

Korda, M. *Power!* New York: Warner Books, 1985.

Miller, R. B., Heiman, S. E., and Tuleja, T. *Strategic Selling.* New York: Warner Books, 1985.

Naisbitt, J., and Aburdene, P. *Re-Inventing the Corporation.* New York: Warner Books, 1985.

Piper, W. *The Little Engine That Could.* New York: Platt & Munk, 1961.

Sloan, A. P. *My Years with General Motors.* New York: Doubleday, 1963.

Srivastva, S., and Associates. *Executive Power: How Executives Influence People and Organizations.* San Francisco: Jossey-Bass, 1986.

Tichy, N. M., and Devanna, M. A. *The Transformational Leader.* New York: Wiley, 1986.

Toffler, A. *Future Shock.* New York: Bantam Books, 1971.

Waterman, R. H., Jr. *The Renewal Factor.* New York: Bantam Books, 1987.

10.   Preparing for Transformation

Lawrence, P. R., and Lorsch, J. W. *Developing Organizations: Diagnosis and Action.* Reading, Mass.: Addison-Wesley, 1969.

Schein, E. H. *Organizational Psychology.* (2nd ed.) Englewood Cliffs, N.J.: Prentice-Hall, 1972.

Senge, P. M. *The Fifth Discipline.* New York: Doubleday Currency, 1990.

Sheldon, A. *Managing Doctors.* Homewood, Ill.: Dow Jones–Irwin, 1986.

11.   Implementing the Renewal Strategy

Beckhard, R. *Organization Development: Strategies and Models.* Reading, Mass.: Addison-Wesley, 1969.

Beckhard, R., and Harris, R. T. *Organizational Transitions: Managing Complex Change.* Reading, Mass.: Addison-Wesley, 1977.

Bennis, W. G. *Organization Development: Its Nature, Origins, and Prospects.* Reading, Mass.: Addison-Wesley, 1969.

Kilmann, R. H. *Beyond the Quick Fix: Managing Five Tracks to Organizational Success.* San Francisco: Jossey-Bass, 1984.

Kirkpatrick, D. L. *How to Manage Change Effectively: Approaches, Methods, and Case Examples.* San Francisco: Jossey-Bass, 1985.

12.   Accelerating the Change Process

Blake, R. R., and Mouton, J. S. *Building a Dynamic Corporation Through Grid Organization Development.* Reading, Mass.: Addison-Wesley, 1969.

Ulrich, D., and Lake, D. *Organizational Capability.* New York: Wiley, 1990.

13. Driving Change with Rewards

Collins, M. *Marva Collins' Way.* (2nd ed.) Los Angeles: J. P. Tarcher, 1990.

Derr, C. B. *Managing the New Careerists: The Diverse Career Success Orientations of Today's Workers.* San Francisco: Jossey-Bass, 1986.

Ford, R. N. *Motivation Through the Work Itself.* New York: AMACOM, 1969.

Gellerman, S. W. *Management by Motivation.* New York: AMACOM, 1968.

LeBoeuf, M. *The Greatest Management Principle in the World.* New York: Berkley, 1985.

McCormack, M. N. *What They Don't Teach You at the Harvard Business School.* New York: Bantam Books, 1984.

Index

311